CW00972813

Type 1 Diabetes Cookbook

100 Quick and Easy Recipes for Type 1 Diabetes

Table of Contents

3

4

Introduction

Type 1 diabetes (T1D) occurs when the body is unable to produce insulin, a hormone produced by the pancreas. Although the exact cause is unknown, it is believed to be a combination of genetics and environment. Today, an estimated 1.25 million people live with T1D in the United States, and 40,000 people are diagnosed every year. T1D results when the body's immune system attacks and destroys its own cells; in this case, it kills the healthy insulin-producing cells. Without insulin from these cells, the body is unable to help sugar (glucose) enter the cells to provide energy.

I wish there were another answer, but currently, management of T1D always requires insulin. Regardless of any changes you implement in your diet, vitamin intake, or lifestyle, if you are diagnosed with T1D, you will need insulin.

Insulin is an amazing hormone produced by the pancreas. The pancreas works to regulate blood sugar, or glucose, levels. It works like this: You eat something, your body digests the foods you eat, and some of that food (mostly carbohydrates but also protein and some fats) converts to glucose, which is the body's primary source of energy. Once glucose is released into the bloodstream, the pancreas responds and releases insulin, which helps move the glucose into our cells for energy. With type 1 diabetes, an outside source of insulin needs to be delivered to do the job; this is typically achieved by injecting insulin or by using an insulin pump. T1D differs from T2D in that in type 2, the body actually produces insulin, but often the insulin that is produced does not work effectively. With T2D, oral medication, non-insulin injectables, and lifestyle changes are the primary treatments

The following dietary guidelines will be helpful to anyone with type 1 diabetes.

Aim for a balanced diet. Seek out carbohydrates that are full of fiber, such as whole grains, fresh fruits, and nonprocessed vegetables. Include fish three times per week, as well as lean meats and calcium-rich protein sources, like tofu and milk. Use healthy fats, such as monounsaturated fat—these include olive and avocado oils, seeds, nuts, and nut butters. Enjoy caffeine and alcohol in moderation, limit simple sugars, and drink plenty of water.

Understand insulin action and meal timing. If you're unclear about how to time your insulin and meals, please discuss this with your diabetes educator. To be effective, insulin and meal timing need to coordinate; this will also help prevent low and high blood sugars.

Read labels. Reading labels is one of the most important things you can do in the grocery store. Become a label-reading pro! In doing so, try not to fall for any misleading claims, like those that read "sugar-free" or "no added sugar." Look at serving sizes and total grams of carbohydrates. Aim for products with at least 3 grams of fiber per 100 calories and less than 5 grams of sugar.

Include healthy proteins. Protein is essential for cell growth and repair. Include healthy, lean proteins, such as fish, tofu, or poultry. You will not take insulin to cover for protein portions unless you are eating unusually large amounts compared to your regular intake.

Carry a simple form of sugar. Keep portable snacks with you, like juice boxes, sports drinks, hard candy, jelly beans, dried fruit, honey, or glucose tablets or gels. You may need them to treat low blood sugars. Even with the best of intentions, low blood sugars can occur, so be prepared by keeping simple sugars on hand.

If you drink alcohol, eat when you do. Surprisingly, alcohol can lower blood sugars. It's always a good idea to eat some form of carbohydrates when you have a cocktail. Talk to your doctor about the best way to manage food, alcohol, and insulin.

Drink plenty of water. Is there any diet that doesn't advocate water? This diet is no different. In fact, it may be even more important for people with diabetes, since people with diabetes are at higher risk for dehydration. Don't wait until you're thirsty, and try to drink 8 to 10 glasses of water throughout the day. Also, limit beverages containing caffeine! Aim for less than 250 milligrams of caffeine daily.

Food List For Type 1 Diabetes

Treatment through the dietary approach is considered the most effective and logical today. Many of the fatal health conditions are now treated only with a well-oriented health diet plan. The same is true for diabetes. With few adjustments in the routine menu, a patient can maintain his glucose levels without the use of medicines. To make this idea work, we need to cut down the direct or high sources of glucose in the food. Here is the complete list of the items which can be taken on a diabetes-friendly diet.

What to Have on A Type 1 Diabetic Diet
Vegetables
Fresh vegetables never cause harm to anyone. So, adding a meal full of vegetables is the best shot for all diabetic patients. But not all vegetables contain the same number of macronutrients. Some vegetables contain a high amount of carbohydrates, so those are not suitable for a diabetic diet. We need to use vegetables which contain a low amount of carbohydrates.

1. Cauliflower
2. Spinach
3. Tomatoes
4. Broccoli
5. Lemons
6. Artichoke
7. Garlic
8. Asparagus
9. Spring onions
10. Onions
11. Ginger etc.

Meat
Meat is not on the red list for the diabetic diet. It is fine to have some meat every now and then for diabetic patients. However certain meat types are better than others. For instance, red meat is not a preferable option for such patients. They should consume white meat more often whether it's seafood or poultry. Healthy options in meat are:

1. All fish, i.e., salmon, halibut, trout, cod, sardine, etc.

2. Scallops
3. Mussels
4. Shrimp
5. Oysters etc.

Fruits

Not all fruits are good for diabetes. To know if the fruit is suitable for this diet, it is important to note its sugar content. Some fruits contain a high number of sugars in the form of sucrose and fructose, and those should be readily avoided. Here is the list of popularly used fruits which can be taken on the diabetic diet:

1. Peaches
2. Nectarines
3. Avocados
4. Apples
5. Berries
6. Grapefruit
7. Kiwi Fruit
8. Bananas
9. Cherries
10. Grapes
11. Orange
12. Pears
13. Plums
14. Strawberries

Nuts and Seeds

Nuts and seeds are perhaps the most enriched edibles, and they contain such a mix of macronutrients which can never harm anyone. So diabetic patients can take the nuts and seeds in their diet without any fear of a glucose spike.

1. Pistachios
2. Sunflower seeds
3. Walnuts
4. Peanuts
5. Pecans
6. Pumpkin seeds
7. Almonds
8. Sesame seeds etc.

Grains

Diabetic patients should also be selective while choosing the right grains for their diet. The idea is to keep the amount of starch as minimum as possible. That is why you won't see any white rice in the list rather it is replaced with more fibrous brown rice.

1. Quinoa
2. Oats
3. Multigrain
4. Whole grains
5. Brown rice
6. Millet
7. Barley
8. Sorghum
9. Tapioca

Fats

Fat intake is the most debated topic as far as the diabetic diet is concerned. As there are diets like ketogenic, which are loaded with fats and still proved effective for diabetic patients. The key is the absence of carbohydrates. In any other situation, the fats are as harmful to people with diabetes as any normal person. Switching to unsaturated fats is a better option.

1. Sesame oil
2. Olive oil
3. Canola oil
4. Grapeseed oil
5. Other vegetable oils
6. Fats extracted from plant sources.

Diary

Any dairy product which directly or indirectly causes a glucose rise in the blood should not be taken on this diet. other than those, all products are good to use. These items include:

1. Skimmed milk
2. Low-fat cheese
3. Eggs
4. Yogurt
5. Trans fat-free margarine or butter

Sugar Alternatives

Since ordinary sugars or sweeteners are strictly forbidden on a diabetic diet. There are artificial varieties that can add sweetness without raising the level of carbohydrates in the meal. These substitutes are:

1. Stevia
2. Xylitol
3. Natvia
4. Swerve
5. Monk fruit
6. Erythritol

Make sure to substitute them with extra care. The sweetness of each sweetener is entirely different from the table sugar, so add each in accordance with the intensity of their flavor. Stevia is the sweetest of them, and it should be used with more care. In place of 1 cup of sugar, a teaspoon of stevia is enough. All other sweeteners are more or less similar to sugar in their intensity of sweetness.

Foods to Avoid

Knowing a general scheme of diet helps a lot, but it is equally important to be well familiar with the items which have to be avoided. With this list, you can make your diet a hundred% sugar-free. There are many other food items which can cause some harm to a diabetic patient as the sugars do. So, let's discuss them in some detail here.

1. Sugars

Sugar is a big NO-GO for a diabetic diet. Once you have diabetes, you would need to say goodbye to all the natural sweeteners which are loaded with carbohydrates. They contain polysaccharides which readily break into glucose after getting into our body. And the list does not only include table sugars but other items like honey and molasses should also be avoided.

1. White sugar
2. Brown sugar
3. Confectionary sugar
4. Honey
5. Molasses
6. Granulated sugar

It is not easy to suddenly stop using sugar. Your mind and your body, will not accept the abrupt change. It is recommended to go for a gradual change. It means start substituting it with low carb substitutes in a small amount, day by day.

2. High Fat Dairy Products

Once you have diabetes, you may get susceptible to a number of other fatal diseases including cardiovascular ones. That is why experts strictly recommend avoiding high-fat food products, especially dairy items. The high amount of fat can make your body insulin resistant. So even when you take insulin, it won't be of any use as the body will not work on it.

3. Saturated Animal Fats

Saturated animal fats are not good for anyone, whether diabetic or normal. So, better avoid using them in general. Whenever you are cooking meat, try to trim off all the excess fat. Cooking oils made out of these saturated fats should be avoided. Keep yourself away from any of the animal origin fats.

4. High Carb Vegetables

Vegetables with more starch are not suitable for diabetes. These veggies can increase the carbohydrate levels of food. So, omit these from the recipes and enjoy the rest of the less starchy vegetables. Some of the high carb vegetables are:

1. Potatoes
2. Sweet potatoes
3. Yams etc.

5. Cholesterol Rich Ingredients

Bad cholesterol or High-density Lipoprotein has the tendency to deposit in different parts of the body and obstructs the flow of blood and the regulation of hormones. That is why food items having high bad cholesterol are not good for diabetes. Such things should be replaced with the ones with low cholesterol.

6. High Sodium Products

Sodium is related to hypertension and blood pressure. Since diabetes is already the result of a hormonal imbalance in the body, in the presence of excess sodium—another imbalance—a fluid imbalance may occur which a diabetic body cannot tolerate. It adds up to already present complications of the disease. So, avoid using food items with a high amount of sodium. Mainly store packed items, processed foods, and salt all contain sodium, and one should avoid them all. Use only the 'Unsalted' variety of food products, whether it's butter, margarine, nuts, or other items.

7. Sugary Drinks

Cola drinks or other similar beverages are filled with sugars. If you had seen different video presentations showing the amount of the sugars present in a single bottle of soda, you would know how dangerous those are for diabetic patients. They can drastically increase the amount of blood glucose level within 30 minutes of drinking. Fortunately, there are many sugar-free varieties available in the drinks which are suitable for diabetic patients.

8. Sugar Syrups and Toppings

A number of syrups available in the markets are made out of nothing but sugar. Maple syrup is one good example. For a diabetic diet, the patient should avoid such sugary syrups and also stay away from the sugar-rich toppings available in the stores. If you want to use them at all, trust yourself and prepare them at home with a sugar-free recipe.

9. Sweet Chocolate and Candies

For diabetic patients, sugar-free chocolates or candies are the best way out. Other processed chocolate bars and sweets are extremely damaging to their health, and all of these should be avoided. You can try and prepare healthy bars and candies at home with sugar-free recipes.

10. Alcohol

Alcohol has the tendency to reduce the rate of our metabolism and take away our appetite, which can render a diabetic patient into a very life-threatening condition. Drink in a very small amount cannot harm the patient, but the regular or constant intake of alcohol is bad for health and glucose levels.

Breakfast

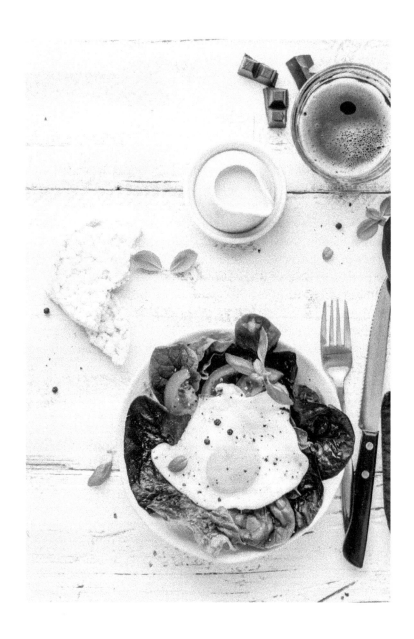

1. Pineapple & Strawberry Smoothie

Preparation Time: 7 minutes
Cooking Time: 0 minute
Servings: 2
Ingredients :

- 1 cup strawberries
- 1 cup pineapple, chopped
- ¾ cup almond milk
- 1 tablespoon almond butter

Directions:

1. Add all **Ingredients** to a blender.
2. Blend until smooth.
3. Add more almond milk until it reaches your desired consistency.
4. Chill before serving.

Nutrition:

- 255 Calories
- 39g Carbohydrate
- 5.6g Protein

2. Green Smoothie

Preparation Time: 12 minutes
Cooking Time: 0 minute
Servings: 2
Ingredients :

- 1 cup vanilla almond milk (unsweetened)
- ¼ ripe avocado, chopped
- 1 cup kale, chopped
- 1 banana
- 2 teaspoons honey
- 1 tablespoon chia seeds
- 1 cup ice cubes

Directions:

1. Combine all the **Ingredients** in a blender.
2. Process until creamy.

Nutrition:

- 343 Calories
- 14.7g Carbohydrate
- 5.9g Protein

3. Spicy Jalapeno Popper Deviled Eggs

Preparation Time: 5 minutes
Cooking Time: 5 minutes
Servings: 4
Ingredients

- 4 large whole eggs, hardboiled
- 2 tablespoons Keto-Friendly mayonnaise
- ¼ cup cheddar cheese, grated
- 2 slices bacon, cooked and crumbled
- 1 jalapeno, sliced

Directions:

1. Cut eggs in half, remove the yolk and put them in bowl
2. Lay egg whites on a platter
3. Mix in remaining **Ingredients** and mash them with the egg yolks
4. Transfer yolk mix back to the egg whites
5. Serve and enjoy!

Nutrition:

- Calories: 176
- Fat: 14g
- Carbohydrates: 0.7g
- Protein: 10g

4. Lovely Porridge

Preparation Time: 15 minutes
Cooking Time: Nil
Servings: 2
Ingredients

- 2 tablespoons coconut flour
- 2 tablespoons vanilla protein powder
- 3 tablespoons Golden Flaxseed meal
- 1 and 1/2 cups almond milk, unsweetened
- Powdered erythritol

Directions:

1. Take a bowl and mix in flaxseed meal, protein powder, coconut flour and mix well
2. Add mix to the saucepan (placed over medium heat)
3. Add almond milk and stir, let the mixture thicken
4. Add your desired amount of sweetener and serve
5. Enjoy!

Nutrition:

- Calories: 259, Fat: 13g
- Carbohydrates: 5g; Protein: 16g

5. Salty Macadamia Chocolate Smoothie

Preparation Time: 5 minutes
Cooking Time: Nil
Servings: 1
Ingredients

- 2 tablespoons macadamia nuts, salted
- 1/3 cup chocolate whey protein powder, low carb
- 1 cup almond milk, unsweetened

Directions:

1. Add the listed **Ingredients** to your blender and blend until you have a smooth mixture
2. Chill and enjoy it!

Nutrition:

- Calories: 165
- Fat: 2g
- Carbohydrates: 1g
- Protein: 12g

6. Basil and Tomato Baked Eggs

Preparation Time: 10 minutes
Cooking Time: 15 minutes
Servings: 4
Ingredients

- 1 garlic clove, minced
- 1 cup canned tomatoes
- ¼ cup fresh basil leaves, roughly chopped
- 1/2 teaspoon chili powder
- 1 tablespoon olive oil
- 4 whole eggs
- Salt and pepper to taste

Directions:

1. Preheat your oven to 375 degrees F
2. Take a small baking dish and grease with olive oil
3. Add garlic, basil, tomatoes chili, olive oil into a dish and stir
4. Crackdown eggs into a dish, keeping space between the two
5. Sprinkle the whole dish with salt and pepper
6. Place in oven and cook for 12 minutes until eggs are set and tomatoes are bubbling
7. Serve with basil on top
8. Enjoy!

Nutrition:

- Calories 235
- Fat: 16g
- Carbohydrates7g
- Protein: 14g

7. Cinnamon and Coconut Porridge

Preparation Time: 5 minutes
Cooking Time: 5 minutes
Servings: 4
Ingredients

- 2 cups of water
- 1 cup 36% heavy cream
- 1/2 cup unsweetened dried coconut, shredded
- 2 tablespoons flaxseed meal
- 1 tablespoon butter
- 1 and 1/2 teaspoon stevia
- 1 teaspoon cinnamon
- Salt to taste
- Toppings as blueberries

Directions:

1. Add the listed **Ingredients** to a small pot, mix well
2. Transfer pot to stove and place it over medium-low heat
3. Bring to mix to a slow boil
4. Stir well and remove the heat
5. Divide the mix into equal servings and let them sit for 10 minutes
6. Top with your desired toppings and enjoy!

Nutrition:

- Calories: 171
- Fat:16g
- Carbohydrates: 6g
- Protein: 2g

8. An Omelet of Swiss chard

Preparation Time: 5 minutes
Cooking Time: 5 minutes
Servings: 4
Ingredients

- 4 eggs, lightly beaten
- 4 cups Swiss chard, sliced
- 2 tablespoons butter
- 1/2 teaspoon garlic salt
- Fresh pepper

Directions:

1. Take a non-stick frying pan and place it over medium-low heat
2. Once the butter melts, add Swiss chard and stir cook for 2 minutes
3. Pour egg into the pan and gently stir them into Swiss chard
4. Season with garlic salt and pepper
5. Cook for 2 minutes
6. Serve and enjoy!

Nutrition:

- Calories: 260
- Fat: 21g
- Carbohydrates: 4g
- Protein: 14g

9. Chipotle Lettuce Chicken

Preparation Time: 10 minutes
Cooking Time: 25 minutes
Servings: 6
Ingredients

- 1 pound chicken breast, cut into strips
- Splash of olive oil
- 1 red onion, finely sliced
- 14 ounces tomatoes

- 1 teaspoon chipotle, chopped
- 1/2 teaspoon cumin
- Pinch of sugar
- Lettuce as needed
- Fresh coriander leaves
- Jalapeno chilies, sliced
- Fresh tomato slices for garnish
- Lime wedges

Directions:
1. Take a non-stick frying pan and place it over medium heat
2. Add oil and heat it up
3. Add chicken and cook until brown
4. Keep the chicken on the side
5. Add tomatoes, sugar, chipotle, cumin to the same pan and simmer for 25 minutes until you have a nice sauce
6. Add chicken into the sauce and cook for 5 minutes
7. Transfer the mix to another place
8. Use lettuce wraps to take a portion of the mixture and serve with a squeeze of lemon
9. Enjoy!

Nutrition:

- Calories: 332
- Fat: 15g
- Carbohydrates: 13g
- Protein: 34g

10. Stylish Chicken-Bacon Wrap

Preparation Time: 5 minutes
Cooking Time: 50 minutes
Servings: 3
Ingredients

- 8 ounces lean chicken breast
- 6 bacon slices
- 3 ounces shredded cheese
- 4 slices ham

Directions:

1. Cut chicken breast into bite-sized portions
2. Transfer shredded cheese onto ham slices
3. Roll up chicken breast and ham slices in bacon slices
4. Take a skillet and place it over medium heat
5. Add olive oil and brown bacon for a while
6. Remove rolls and transfer to your oven
7. Bake for 45 minutes at 325 degrees F
8. Serve and enjoy!

Nutrition:

- Calories: 275
- Fat: 11g
- Carbohydrates: 0.5g
- Protein: 40g

11. Healthy Cottage Cheese Pancakes

Preparation Time: 10 minutes
Cooking Time: 15
Servings: 1
Ingredients :

- 1/2 cup of Cottage cheese (low-fat)
- 1/3 cup (approx. 2 egg whites) Egg whites
- ¼ cup of Oats
- 1 teaspoon of Vanilla extract
- Olive oil cooking spray
- 1 tablespoon of Stevia (raw)
- Berries or sugar-free jam (optional)

Directions:

1. Begin by taking a food blender and adding in the egg whites and cottage cheese. Also add in the vanilla extract, a pinch of stevia, and oats. Palpitate until the consistency is well smooth.
2. Get a nonstick pan and oil it nicely with the cooking spray. Position the pan on low heat.

3. After it has been heated, scoop out half of the batter and pour it on the pan. Cook for about 21/2 minutes on each side.
4. Position the cooked pancakes on a serving plate and cover with sugar-free jam or berries.

Nutrition:

- Calories: 205

calories per serving

- Fat 1.5 g
- Protein 24.5 g
- Carbohydrates 19 g

12. Avocado Lemon Toast

Preparation Time: 10 minutes
Cooking Time: 13 minutes
Servings: 2
Ingredients :
- Whole-grain bread – 2 slices
- Fresh cilantro (chopped) – 2 tablespoons
- Lemon zest – ¼ teaspoon
- Fine sea salt – 1 pinch

Directions:
1. Begin by getting a medium-sized mixing bowl and adding in the avocado. Make use of a fork to crush it properly.
2. Then, add in the cilantro, lemon zest, lemon juice, sea salt, and cayenne pepper. Mix well until combined.
3. Toast the bread slices in a toaster until golden brown. It should take about 3 minutes.
4. Top the toasted bread slices with the avocado mixture and finalize by drizzling with chia seeds.

Nutrition:

- Calories: 72

calories per serving

- Protein 3.6 g
- Avocado 1/2
- Fresh lemon juice 1 teaspoon
- Cayenne pepper 1 pinch
- Chia seeds ¼ teaspoon
- Fat 1.2 g
- Carbohydrates 11.6 g

13. Healthy Baked Eggs

Preparation Time: 10 minutes
Cooking Time: 1 hour
Servings: 6
Ingredients :

- Olive oil – 1 tablespoon
- Garlic – 2 cloves
- Eggs – 8 larges
- Sea salt – 1/2 teaspoon
- Shredded mozzarella cheese (medium-fat) – 3 cups
- Olive oil spray
- Onion (chopped) – 1 medium
- Spinach leaves – 8 ounces
- Half-and-half – 1 cup
- Black pepper – 1 teaspoon
- Feta cheese – 1/2 cup

Directions:

1. Begin by heating the oven to 375F.
2. Get a glass baking dish and grease it with olive oil spray. Arrange aside.
3. Now take a nonstick pan and pour in the olive oil. Position the pan on allows heat and allows it heat.
4. Immediately you are done, toss in the garlic, spinach, and onion. Prepare for about 5 minutes. Arrange aside.

5. You can now Get a large mixing bowl and add in the half, eggs, pepper, and salt. Whisk thoroughly to combine.
6. Put in the feta cheese and chopped mozzarella cheese (reserve 1/2 cup of mozzarella cheese for later).
7. Put the egg mixture and prepared spinach to the prepared glass baking dish. Blend well to combine. Drizzle the reserved cheese over the top.
8. Bake the egg mix for about 45 minutes.
9. Extract the baking dish from the oven and allow it to stand for 10 minutes.
10. Dice and serve!

Nutrition:

- Calories: 323

calories per serving

- Fat 22.3 g
- Protein 22.6 g
- Carbohydrates 7.9 g

14. Quick Low-Carb Oatmeal

Preparation Time: 10 minutes
Cooking Time: 15 minutes
Servings: 2
Ingredients :

- Almond flour – 1/2 cup
- Flax meal – 2 tablespoons
- Cinnamon (ground) – 1 teaspoon
- Almond milk (unsweetened) – 11/2 cups
- Salt – as per taste
- Chia seeds – 2 tablespoons
- Liquid stevia – 10 – 15 drops
- Vanilla extract – 1 teaspoon

Directions:

1. Begin by taking a large mixing bowl and adding in the coconut flour, almond flour, ground cinnamon, flax seed powder, and chia seeds. Mix properly to combine.
2. Position a stockpot on a low heat and add in the dry **Ingredients** . Also add in the liquid stevia, vanilla extract, and almond milk. Mix well to combine.
3. Prepare the flour and almond milk for about 4 minutes. Add salt if needed.
4. Move the oatmeal to a serving bowl and top with nuts, seeds, and pure and neat berries.

Nutrition:

calories per serving

- Protein 11.7 g
- Fat 24.3 g
- Carbohydrates – 16.7 g

15. Tofu and Vegetable Scramble

Preparation Time: 10 minutes
Cooking Time: 15 minutes
Servings: 2
Ingredients :

- Firm tofu (drained) – 16 ounces
- Sea salt – 1/2 teaspoon
- Garlic powder – 1 teaspoon
- Fresh coriander – for garnishing
- Red onion – 1/2 medium
- Cumin powder – 1 teaspoon
- Lemon juice – for topping
- Green bell pepper – 1 medium
- Garlic powder – 1 teaspoon
- Fresh coriander – for garnishing
- Red onion – 1/2 medium
- Cumin powder – 1 teaspoon
- Lemon juice – for topping

Directions:

1. Begin by preparing the **Ingredients** . For this, you are to extract the seeds of the tomato and green bell pepper. Shred the onion, bell pepper, and tomato into small cubes.
2. Get a small mixing bowl and position the fairly hard tofu inside it. Make use of your hands to break the fairly hard tofu. Arrange aside.
3. Get a nonstick pan and add in the onion, tomato, and bell pepper. Mix and cook for about 3 minutes.
4. Put the somewhat hard crumbled tofu to the pan and combine well.

5. Get a small bowl and put in the water, turmeric, garlic powder, cumin powder, and chili powder. Combine well and stream it over the tofu and vegetable mixture.
6. Allow the tofu and vegetable crumble cook with seasoning for 5 minutes. Continuously stir so that the pan is not holding the **Ingredients** . Drizzle the tofu scramble with chili flakes and salt. Combine well.
7. Transfer the prepared scramble to a serving bowl and give it a proper spray of lemon juice.
8. Finalize by garnishing with pure and neat coriander. Serve while hot!

Nutrition:

- Calories: 238

calories per serving

- Carbohydrates 16.6 g
- Fat 11 g

16. Cantaloupe Smoothie
Preparation Time: 11 minutes
Cooking Time: 0 minute
Serving: 2
Ingredients :
- ¾ cup carrot juice
- 4 cups cantaloupe, sliced into cubes

- Pinch of salt
- Frozen melon balls
- Fresh basil

Directions:

1. Add the carrot juice and cantaloupe cubes to a blender. Sprinkle with salt.
2. Process until smooth.
3. Transfer to a bowl.
4. Chill in the refrigerator for at least 30 minutes.
5. Top with the frozen melon balls and basil before serving.

Nutrition:

- 135 Calories
- 31g Carbohydrate
- 3.4g Protein

17. Berry Smoothie with Mint

Preparation Time: 7 minutes
Cooking Time: 0 minute
Serving: 2
Ingredients :
- ¼ cup orange juice
- ½ cup blueberries
- ½ cup blackberries
- 1 cup reduced-fat plain kefir
- 1 tablespoon honey
- 2 tablespoons fresh mint leaves

Directions:

1. Add all the **Ingredients** to a blender.
2. Blend until smooth.

Nutrition:

- 137 Calories
- 27g Carbohydrate ; 6g Protein

Lunch

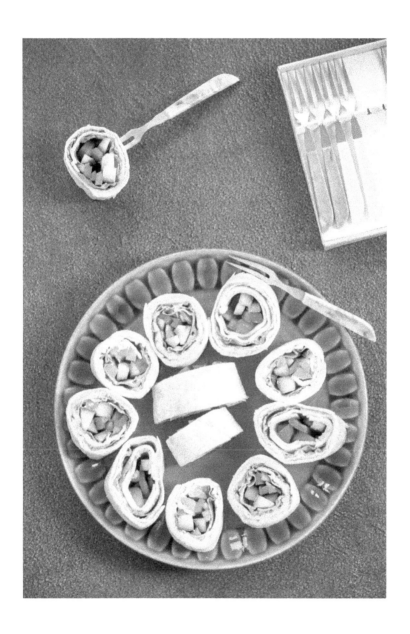

18. Berry Apple Cider

Preparation Time: 15 minutes
Cooking Time: 3 hours
Servings: 3
Ingredients

- 4 cinnamon sticks, cut into 1-inch pieces
- 1½ teaspoons whole cloves
- 4 cups apple cider
- 4 cups low-calorie cranberry-raspberry juice drink
- 1 medium apple

Direction

1. To make the spice bag, cut out a 6-inch square from double thick, pure cotton cheesecloth. Put in the cloves and cinnamon, then bring the corners up, tie it closed using a clean kitchen string that is pure cotton.
2. In a 3 1/2- 5-quart slow cooker, combine cranberry-raspberry juice, apple cider, and the spice bag.
3. Cook while covered over low heat setting for around 4-6 hours or on a high heat setting for 2-2 1/2 hours.
4. Throw out the spice bag. Serve right away or keep it warm while covered on friendly or low-heat setting up to 2 hours, occasionally stirring. Garnish each serving with apples (thinly sliced).

Nutrition

- 89 Calories
- 22g Carbohydrate
- 19g Sugar

19. Brunswick Stew

Preparation Time: 10 minutes
Cooking Time: 45 minutes
Servings: 3
Ingredients

- 4 ounces diced salt pork
- 2 pounds chicken parts
- 8 cups water
- 3 potatoes, cubed
- 3 onions, chopped
- 1 (28 ounce) can whole peeled tomatoes
- 2 cups canned whole kernel corn
- 1 (10 ounce) package frozen lima beans
- 1 tablespoon Worcestershire sauce
- 1/2 teaspoon salt
- 1/4 teaspoon ground black pepper

Direction

1. Mix and boil water, chicken and salt pork in a big pot on high heat. Lower heat to low. Cover then simmer until chicken is tender for 45 minutes.
2. Take out chicken. Let cool until easily handled. Take meat out. Throw out bones and skin. Chop meat to bite-sized pieces. Put back in the soup.
3. Add ground black pepper, salt, Worcestershire sauce, lima beans, corn, tomatoes, onions and potatoes. Mix well. Stir well and simmer for 1 hour, uncovered.

Nutrition

- 368 Calories
- 25.9g Carbohydrate
- 27.9g Protein

20. Buffalo Chicken Salads

Preparation Time: 7 minutes
Cooking Time: 3 hours
Servings: 5
Ingredients

- 1½ pounds chicken breast halves
- ½ cup Wing Time® Buffalo chicken sauce
- 4 teaspoons cider vinegar
- 1 teaspoon Worcestershire sauce
- 1 teaspoon paprika
- 1/3 cup light mayonnaise
- 2 tablespoons fat-free milk
- 2 tablespoons crumbled blue cheese
- 2 romaine hearts, chopped
- 1 cup whole grain croutons
- ½ cup very thinly sliced red onion

Direction

1. Place chicken in a 2-quarts slow cooker. Mix Worcestershire sauce, 2 teaspoons of vinegar and Buffalo sauce in a small bowl; pour over chicken. Dust with paprika. Close and cook for 3 hours on low-heat setting.
2. Mix the leftover 2 teaspoons of vinegar with milk and light mayonnaise together in a small bowl at serving time; mix in blue cheese. While chicken is still in the slow cooker, pull meat into bite-sized pieces using two forks.
3. Split the romaine among 6 dishes. Spoon sauce and chicken over lettuce. Pour with blue cheese dressing then add red onion slices and croutons on top.

Nutrition

- 274 Calories
- 11g Carbohydrate
- 2g Fiber

21. Cacciatore Style Chicken

Preparation Time: 10 minutes
Cooking Time: 4 hours
Servings: 6
Ingredients

- 2 cups sliced fresh mushrooms
- 1 cup sliced celery
- 1 cup chopped carrot
- 2 medium onions, cut into wedges
- 1 green, yellow, or red sweet peppers
- 4 cloves garlic, minced
- 12 chicken drumsticks
- ½ cup chicken broth
- ¼ cup dry white wine
- 2 tablespoons quick-cooking tapioca
- 2 bay leaves
- 1 teaspoon dried oregano, crushed
- 1 teaspoon sugar
- ½ teaspoon salt
- ¼ teaspoon pepper
- 1 (14.5 ounce) can diced tomatoes
- 1/3 cup tomato paste
- Hot cooked pasta or rice

Direction

1. Mix garlic, sweet pepper, onions, carrot, celery and mushrooms in a 5- or 6-qt. slow cooker. Cover veggies with the chicken. Add pepper, salt, sugar, oregano, bay leaves, tapioca, wine and broth.
2. Cover. Cook for 3–3 1/2 hours on high-heat setting.
3. Take chicken out; keep warm. Discard bay leaves. Turn to high-heat setting if using low-heat setting. Mix tomato paste and undrained tomatoes in. Cover. Cook on high-heat setting for 15 more minutes. **Servings:** Put veggie mixture on top of pasta and chicken.

Nutrition

- 324 Calories
- 7g Sugar:
- 35g Carbohydrate

22. Carnitas Tacos

Preparation Time: 10 minutes
Cooking Time: 5 hours
Servings: 4
Ingredients

- 3 to 3½-pound bone-in pork shoulder roast
- ½ cup chopped onion
- 1/3 cup orange juice
- 1 tablespoon ground cumin
- 1½ teaspoons kosher salt
- 1 teaspoon dried oregano, crushed
- ¼ teaspoon cayenne pepper
- 1 lime
- 2 (5.3 ounce) containers plain low-fat Greek yogurt
- 1 pinch kosher salt
- 16 (6 inch) soft yellow corn tortillas, such as Mission® brand
- 4 leaves green cabbage, quartered
- 1 cup very thinly sliced red onion
- 1 cup salsa (optional)

Direction

1. Take off meat from the bone; throw away bone. Trim meat fat. Slice meat into 2 to 3-inch pieces; put in a slow cooker of 3 1/2 or 4-quart in size. Mix in cayenne, oregano, salt, cumin, orange juice and onion.
2. Cover and cook for 4 to 5 hours on high. Take out meat from the cooker. Shred meat with two forks. Mix in enough cooking liquid to moisten.

3. Take out 1 teaspoon zest (put aside) for lime crema, squeeze 2 tablespoons lime juice. Mix dash salt, yogurt, and lime juice in a small bowl.
4. Serve lime crema, salsa (if wished), red onion and cabbage with meat in tortillas. Scatter with lime zest.

Nutrition

- 301 Calories
- 28g Carbohydrate
- 7g Sugar

23. Chicken Chili

Preparation Time: 6 minutes
Cooking Time: 1 hour
Servings: 4
Ingredients
- 3 tablespoons vegetable oil
- 2 cloves garlic, minced
- 1 green bell pepper, chopped
- 1 onion, chopped
- 1 stalk celery, sliced
- 1/4-pound mushrooms, chopped
- 1-pound chicken breast
- 1 tablespoon chili powder
- 1 teaspoon dried oregano
- 1 teaspoon ground cumin
- 1/2 teaspoon paprika
- 1/2 teaspoon cocoa powder
- 1/4 teaspoon salt
- One pinch of crushed red pepper flakes
- One pinch ground black pepper
- 1 (14.5 oz) can tomatoes with juice
- 1 (19 oz) can kidney beans

Direction

1. Fill two tablespoons of oil into a big skillet and heat it at moderate heat. Add mushrooms, celery, onion, bell pepper, and garlic, sautéing for 5 minutes. Put it to one side.
2. Insert the leftover one tablespoon of oil into the skillet. At high heat, cook the chicken until browned and its exterior turns firm. Transfer the vegetable mixture back into the skillet.
3. Stir in ground black pepper, hot pepper flakes, salt, cocoa powder, paprika, oregano, cumin, and chili powder. Continue stirring for several minutes to avoid burning. Pour in the beans and tomatoes, lead the entire mixture to a boiling point, and then adjust the setting to low heat. Place a lid on the skillet and leave it simmering for 15 minutes. Uncover the skillet and leave it simmering for another 15 minutes.

Nutrition

- 308 Calories
- 25.9g Carbohydrate
- 29g Protein

24. Chicken Vera Cruz

Preparation Time: 7 minutes
Cooking Time: 10 hours
Servings: 5
Ingredients

- One medium onion, cut into wedges
- 1-pound yellow-skin potatoes
- Six skinless, boneless chicken thighs
- 2 (14.5 oz.) cans of no-salt-added diced tomatoes
- 1 fresh jalapeño chili pepper
- Two tablespoons Worcestershire sauce
- One tablespoon chopped garlic
- One teaspoon dried oregano, crushed
- ¼ teaspoon ground cinnamon
- 1/8 teaspoon ground cloves

- ½ cup snipped fresh parsley
- ¼ cup chopped pimiento-stuffed green olives

Direction

1. Put the onion in a 3 1/2- or 4-quart slow cooker. Place chicken thighs and potatoes on top. Drain and discard juices from a can of tomatoes. Stir undrained and drained tomatoes, cloves, cinnamon, oregano, garlic, Worcestershire sauce and jalapeño pepper together in a bowl. Pour over all in the cooker.

2. Cook with a cover for 10 hours on low-heat setting.
3. To make the topping: Stir chopped pimiento-stuffed green olives and snipped fresh parsley together in a small bowl. Drizzle the topping over each serving of chicken.

Nutrition

- 228 Calories
- 9g Sugar
- 25g Carbohydrate

25. Chicken and Cornmeal Dumplings

Preparation Time: 8 minutes
Cooking Time: 8 hours
Servings: 4
Ingredients
Chicken and Vegetable Filling

- 2 medium carrots, thinly sliced
- 1 stalk celery, thinly sliced
- 1/3 cup corn kernels
- ½ of a medium onion, thinly sliced
- 2 cloves garlic, minced
- 1 teaspoon snipped fresh rosemary
- ¼ teaspoon ground black pepper
- 2 chicken thighs, skinned

- 1 cup reduced sodium chicken broth
- ½ cup fat-free milk
- 1 tablespoon all-purpose flour

Cornmeal Dumplings
- ¼ cup flour
- ¼ cup cornmeal
- ½ teaspoon baking powder
- 1 egg white
- 1 tablespoon fat-free milk
- 1 tablespoon canola oil

Direction

1. Mix 1/4 teaspoon pepper, carrots, garlic, celery, rosemary, corn, and onion in a 1 1/2 or 2-quart slow cooker. Place chicken on top. Pour the broth atop mixture in the cooker.
2. Close and cook on low-heat for 7 to 8 hours.
3. If cooking with the low-heat setting, switch to high-heat setting (or if heat setting is not available, continue to cook). Place the chicken onto a cutting board and let to cool slightly. Once cool enough to handle, chop off chicken from bones and get rid of the bones. Chop the chicken and place back into the mixture in cooker. Mix flour and milk in a small bowl until smooth. Stir into the mixture in cooker.
4. Drop the Cornmeal Dumplings dough into 4 mounds atop hot chicken mixture using two spoons. Cover and cook for 20 to 25 minutes more or until a toothpick come out clean when inserted into a dumpling. (Avoid lifting lid when cooking.) Sprinkle each of the serving with coarse pepper if desired.
5. Mix together 1/2 teaspoon baking powder, 1/4 cup flour, a dash of salt and 1/4 cup cornmeal in a medium bowl. Mix 1 tablespoon canola oil, 1 egg white and 1 tablespoon fat-free milk in a small bowl. Pour the egg mixture into the flour mixture. Mix just until moistened.

Nutrition

- 369 Calories
- 9g Sugar
- 47g Carbohydrate

26. Chicken and Pepperoni

Preparation Time: 4 minutes
Cooking Time: 4 hours
Servings: 5
Ingredients

- 3½ to 4 pounds meaty chicken pieces
- 1/8 teaspoon salt
- 1/8 teaspoon black pepper
- 2 ounces sliced turkey pepperoni
- ¼ cup sliced pitted ripe olives
- ½ cup reduced-sodium chicken broth
- 1 tablespoon tomato paste
- 1 teaspoon dried Italian seasoning, crushed
- ½ cup shredded part-skim mozzarella cheese (2 ounces)

Direction

1. Put chicken into a 3 1/2 to 5-qt. slow cooker. Sprinkle pepper and salt on the chicken. Slice pepperoni slices in half. Put olives and pepperoni into the slow cooker. In a small bowl, blend Italian seasoning, tomato paste and chicken broth together. Transfer the mixture into the slow cooker.
2. Cook with a cover for 3-3 1/2 hours on high.
3. Transfer the olives, pepperoni and chicken onto a serving platter with a slotted spoon. Discard the cooking liquid. Sprinkle cheese over the chicken. Use foil to loosely cover and allow to sit for 5 minutes to melt the cheese.

Nutrition

- 243 Calories
- 1g Carbohydrate
- 41g Protein

27. Chicken and Sausage Gumbo

Preparation Time: 6 minutes
Cooking Time: 4 hours
Servings: 5
Ingredients

- 1/3 cup all-purpose flour
- 1 (14 ounce) can reduced-sodium chicken broth
- 2 cups chicken breast
- 8 ounces smoked turkey sausage links
- 2 cups sliced fresh okra
- 1 cup water
- 1 cup coarsely chopped onion
- 1 cup sweet pepper
- ½ cup sliced celery
- 4 cloves garlic, minced
- 1 teaspoon dried thyme
- ½ teaspoon ground black pepper
- ¼ teaspoon cayenne pepper
- 3 cups hot cooked brown rice

Direction

1. To make the roux: Cook the flour upon a medium heat in a heavy medium-sized saucepan, stirring periodically, for roughly 6 minutes or until the flour browns. Take off the heat and slightly cool, then slowly stir in the broth. Cook the roux until it bubbles and thickens up.
2. Pour the roux in a 3 1/2- or 4-quart slow cooker, then add in cayenne pepper, black pepper, thyme, garlic, celery, sweet pepper, onion, water, okra, sausage, and chicken.
3. Cook the soup covered on a high setting for 3 - 3 1/2 hours. Take the fat off the top and serve atop hot cooked brown rice.

Nutrition

- 230 Calories
- 3g Sugar
- 19g Protein

28. Chicken, Barley, and Leek Stew

Preparation Time: 10 minutes
Cooking Time: 3 hours
Servings: 2
Ingredients

- 1-pound chicken thighs
- 1 tablespoon olive oil
- 1 (49 ounce) can reduced-sodium chicken broth
- 1 cup regular barley (not quick-cooking)
- 2 medium leeks, halved lengthwise and sliced
- 2 medium carrots, thinly sliced
- 1½ teaspoons dried basil or Italian seasoning, crushed
- ¼ teaspoon cracked black pepper

Direction

1. In the big skillet, cook the chicken in hot oil till becoming brown on all sides. In the 4-5-qt. slow cooker, whisk the pepper, dried basil, carrots, leeks, barley, chicken broth and chicken.
2. Keep covered and cooked over high heat setting for 2 – 2.5 hours or till the barley softens. As you wish, drizzle with the parsley or fresh basil prior to serving.

Nutrition

- 248 Calories
- 6g Fiber
- 27g Carbohydrate

29. Cider Pork Stew

Preparation Time: 9 minutes
Cooking Time: 12 hours
Servings: 3
Ingredients

- 2 pounds pork shoulder roast
- 3 medium cubed potatoes
- 3 medium carrots
- 2 medium onions, sliced
- 1 cup coarsely chopped apple

- ½ cup coarsely chopped celery
- 3 tablespoons quick-cooking tapioca
- 2 cups apple juice
- 1 teaspoon salt
- 1 teaspoon caraway seeds
- ¼ teaspoon black pepper

Direction

1. Chop the meat into 1-in. cubes. In the 3.5- 5.5 qt. slow cooker, mix the tapioca, celery, apple, onions, carrots, potatoes and meat. Whisk in pepper, caraway seeds, salt and apple juice.
2. Keep covered and cook over low heat setting for 10-12 hours. If you want, use the celery leaves to decorate each of the servings.

Nutrition

- 244 Calories
- 5g Fiber
- 33g Carbohydrate

30. Creamy Chicken Noodle Soup

Preparation Time: 7 minutes
Cooking Time: 8 hours
Servings: 4
Ingredients

- 1 (32 fluid ounce) container reduced-sodium chicken broth
- 3 cups water
- 2½ cups chopped cooked chicken
- 3 medium carrots, sliced
- 3 stalks celery
- 1½ cups sliced fresh mushrooms
- ¼ cup chopped onion
- 1½ teaspoons dried thyme, crushed
- ¾ teaspoon garlic-pepper seasoning
- 3 ounces reduced-fat cream cheese (Neufchâtel), cut up

- 2 cups dried egg noodles

Direction

1. Mix together the garlic-pepper seasoning, thyme, onion, mushrooms, celery, carrots, chicken, water and broth in a 5 to 6-quart slow cooker.
2. Put cover and let it cook for 6-8 hours on low-heat setting.
3. Increase to high-heat setting if you are using low-heat setting. Mix in the cream cheese until blended. Mix in uncooked noodles. Put cover and let it cook for an additional 20-30 minutes or just until the noodles become tender.

Nutrition

- 170 Calories
- 3g Sugar
- 2g Fiber

31. Cuban Pulled Pork Sandwich

Preparation Time: 6 minutes
Cooking Time: 5 hours
Servings: 5
Ingredients

- 1 teaspoon dried oregano, crushed
- ¾ teaspoon ground cumin
- ½ teaspoon ground coriander
- ¼ teaspoon salt
- ¼ teaspoon black pepper
- ¼ teaspoon ground allspice
- 1 2 to 2½-pound boneless pork shoulder roast
- 1 tablespoon olive oil
- Nonstick cooking spray
- 2 cups sliced onions
- 2 green sweet peppers, cut into bite-size strips
- ½ to 1 fresh jalapeño pepper
- 4 cloves garlic, minced

- ¼ cup orange juice
- ¼ cup lime juice
- 6 heart-healthy wheat hamburger buns, toasted
- 2 tablespoons jalapeño mustard

Direction

1. Mix allspice, oregano, black pepper, cumin, salt, and coriander together in a small bowl. Press each side of the roast into the spice mixture. On medium-high heat, heat oil in a big non-stick pan; put in roast. Cook for 5mins until both sides of the roast is light brown, turn the roast one time.
2. Using a cooking spray, grease a 3 1/2 or 4qt slow cooker; arrange the garlic, onions, jalapeno, and green peppers in a layer. Pour in lime juice and orange juice. Slice the roast if needed to fit inside the cooker; put on top of the vegetables covered or 4 1/2-5hrs on high heat setting.
3. Move roast to a cutting board using a slotted spoon. Drain the cooking liquid and keep the jalapeno, green peppers, and onions. Shred the roast with 2 forks then place it back in the cooker. Remove fat from the liquid. Mix half cup of cooking liquid and reserved vegetables into the cooker. Pour in more cooking liquid if desired. Discard the remaining cooking liquid.
4. Slather mustard on rolls. Split the meat between the bottom roll halves. Add avocado on top if desired. Place the roll tops to sandwiches.

Nutrition

- 379 Calories
- 32g Carbohydrate
- 4g Fiber

32. Lemony Salmon Burgers

Preparation Time: 10 Minutes
Cooking Time: 10 Minutes
Servings: 4
Ingredients

- 2 (3-oz) cans boneless, skinless pink salmon
- 1/4 cup panko breadcrumbs
- 4 tsp. lemon juice
- 1/4 cup red bell pepper
- 1/4 cup sugar-free yogurt
- 1 egg
- 2 (1.5-oz) whole wheat hamburger toasted buns

Directions

1. Mix drained and flaked salmon, finely-chopped bell pepper, panko breadcrumbs.
2. Combine 2 tbsp. cup sugar-free yogurt, 3 tsp. fresh lemon juice, and egg in a bowl. Shape mixture into 2 (3-inch) patties, bake on the skillet over medium heat 4 to 5 Minutes per side.
3. Stir together 2 tbsp. sugar-free yogurt and 1 tsp. lemon juice; spread over bottom halves of buns.
4. Top each with 1 patty, and cover with bun tops.
5. This dish is very mouth-watering!

Nutrition:

- Calories 131
- Protein 12
- Fat 1 g
- Carbs 19 g

33. Caprese Turkey Burgers

Preparation Time 10 Minutes
Cooking Time: 10 Minutes
Servings: 4
Ingredients

- 1/2 lb. 93% lean ground turkey
- 2 (1,5-oz) whole wheat hamburger buns (toasted)

- 1/4 cup shredded mozzarella cheese (part-skim)
- 1 egg
- 1 big tomato
- 1 small clove garlic
- 4 large basil leaves
- 1/8 tsp. salt
- 1/8 tsp. pepper

Directions

1. Combine turkey, white egg, Minced garlic, salt, and pepper (mix until combined);
2. Shape into 2 cutlets. Put cutlets into a skillet; cook 5 to 7 Minutes per side.
3. Top cutlets properly with cheese and sliced tomato at the end of cooking.
4. Put 1 cutlet on the bottom of each bun.
5. Top each patty with 2 basil leaves. Cover with bun tops.

Nutrition:

- Calories 180
- Protein 7 g
- Fat 4 g
- Carbs 20 g

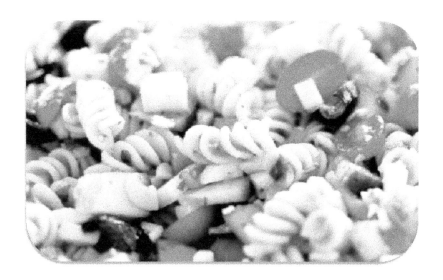

34. Pasta Salad

Preparation Time: 15 Minutes
Cooking Time: 15 Minutes
Servings: 4
Ingredients

- 8 oz. whole-wheat pasta
- 2 tomatoes
- 1 (5-oz) pkg spring mix
- 9 slices bacon
- 1/3 cup mayonnaise (reduced-fat)
- 1 tbsp. Dijon mustard
- 3 tbsp. apple cider vinegar
- 1/4 tsp. salt
- 1/2 tsp. pepper

Directions
1. Cook pasta.
2. Chilled pasta, chopped tomatoes and spring mix in a bowl.
3. Crumble cooked bacon over pasta.
4. Combine mayonnaise, mustard, vinegar, salt and pepper in a small bowl.
5. Pour dressing over pasta, stirring to coat.

Nutrition:

- Calories 200
- Protein 15 g
- Fat 3 g
- Carbs 6 g

35. Ground Turkey Salad

Preparation Time: 10 minutes
Cooking Time: 35 minutes
Servings: 6
Ingredients :

- 1 lb. lean ground turkey
- 1/2 inch ginger, minced
- 2 garlic cloves, minced
- 1 onion, chopped
- 1 tbsp. olive oil
- 1 bag lettuce leaves (for serving)
- ¼ cup fresh cilantro, chopped
- 2 tsp. coriander powder
- 1 tsp. red chili powder
- 1 tsp. turmeric powder
- Salt to taste
- 4 cups water
- Dressing:
- 2 tbsp. fat free yogurt
- 1 tbsp. sour cream, non-fat
- 1 tbsp. low fat mayonnaise
- 1 lemon, juiced
- 1 tsp. red chili flakes
- Salt and pepper to taste

Directions:

1. In a skillet sauté the garlic and ginger in olive oil for 1 minute. Add onion and season with salt. Cook for 10 minutes over medium heat.
2. Add the ground turkey and sauté for 3 more minutes. Add the spices (turmeric, red chili powder and coriander powder).
3. Add 4 cups water and cook for 30 minutes, covered.
4. Prepare the dressing by combining yogurt, sour cream, mayo, lemon juice, chili flakes, salt and pepper.
5. To serve arrange the salad leaves on serving plates and place the cooked ground turkey on them. Top with dressing.

Nutrition:

- Carbohydrates: 9.1
- Protein: 17.8 g
- Total sugars: 2.5 g
- Calories: 176

36. Everyday Salad

Preparation Time: 10 minutes
Cooking Time: 40 minutes
Servings: 6
Ingredients :
- 5 halved mushrooms
- 6 halved Cherry (Plum) Tomatoes
- 6 rinsed Lettuce Leaves
- 10 olives
- ½ chopped cucumber
- Juice from ½ Key Lime
- 1 teaspoon olive oil
- Pure Sea Salt

Directions:
1. Tear rinsed lettuce leaves into medium pieces and put them in a medium salad bowl.
2. Add mushrooms halves, chopped cucumber, olives and cherry tomato halves into the bowl. Mix well. Pour olive and Key Lime juice over salad.
3. Add pure sea salt to taste. Mix it all till it is well combined.

Nutrition:

- Calories: 88
- Carbohydrates: 11g
- Fat: .5g
- Protein: .8g

37. Super-Seedy Salad with Tahini Dressing

Preparation Time: 10 minutes
Cooking Time: 0 minutes
Servings: 1-2
Ingredients :
- 1 slice stale sourdough, torn into chunks
- 50g mixed seeds
- 1 tsp. cumin seeds
- 1 tsp. coriander seeds
- 50g baby kale
- 75g long-stemmed broccoli, blanched for a few minutes then roughly chopped
- ½ red onion, thinly sliced
- 100g cherry tomatoes, halved
- ½ a small bunch flat-leaf parsley, torn

DRESSING
- 100ml natural yogurt
- 1 tbsp. tahini
- 1 lemon, juiced

Directions:

1. Heat the oven to 200°C/fan 180°C/gas 6. Put the bread into a food processor and pulse into very rough breadcrumbs. Put into a bowl with the mixed seeds and spices, season, and spray well with oil. Tip onto a non-stick baking tray and roast for 15-20 minutes, stirring and tossing regularly, until deep golden brown.
2. Whisk together the dressing **Ingredients** , some seasoning and a splash of water in a large bowl. Tip the baby kale, broccoli, red onion, cherry tomatoes and flat-leaf parsley into the dressing, and mix well. Divide between 2 plates and top with the crispy breadcrumbs and seeds.

Nutrition:

- Calories: 78
- Carbohydrates: 6 g
- Fat: 2g
- Protein: 1.5g

38. Vegetable Salad

Preparation Time: 10 minutes
Cooking Time: 0 minutes
Servings: 1-2
Ingredients :

- 4 cups each of raw spinach and romaine lettuce
- 2 cups each of cherry tomatoes, sliced cucumber, chopped baby carrots and chopped red, orange and yellow bell pepper
- 1 cup each of chopped broccoli, sliced yellow squash, zucchini and cauliflower.

Directions:
1. Wash all these vegetables.
2. Mix in a large mixing bowl and top off with a non-fat or low-fat dressing of your choice.

Nutrition:

- Calories: 48
- Carbohydrates: 11g
- Protein: 3g

39. Greek Salad

Preparation Time: 10 minutes
Cooking Time: 0 minutes
Servings: 1-2
Ingredients :

- 1 Romaine head, torn in bits
- 1 cucumber sliced
- 1 pint cherry tomatoes, halved
- 1 green pepper, thinly sliced
- 1 onion sliced into rings
- 1 cup kalamata olives
- 1 ½ cups feta cheese, crumbled
- For dressing combine:
- 1 cup olive oil
- 1/4 cup lemon juice
- 2 tsp. oregano
- Salt and pepper

Directions:
1. Lay **Ingredients** on plate.
2. Drizzle dressing over salad

Nutrition:

- Calories: 107
- Carbohydrates: 18g
- Fat: 1.2 g
- Protein: 1g

40. Alkaline Spring Salad

Preparation Time: 10 minutes
Cooking Time: 0 minutes
Servings: 1-2
Ingredients :

- 4 cups seasonal approved greens of your choice
- 1 cup cherry tomatoes
- 1/4 cup walnuts
- 1/4 cup approved herbs of your choice
- For the dressing:
- 3-4 key limes
- 1 tbsp. of homemade raw sesame
- Sea salt and cayenne pepper

Directions:

1. First, get the juice of the key limes. In a small bowl, whisk together the key lime juice with the homemade raw sesame "tahini" butter. Add sea salt and cayenne pepper, to taste.
2. Cut the cherry tomatoes in half.
3. In a large bowl, combine the greens, cherry tomatoes , and herbs. Pour the dressing on top and "massage" with your hands.
4. Let the greens soak up the dressing. Add more sea salt, cayenne pepper, and herbs on top if you wish. Enjoy!

Nutrition:

- Calories: 77
- Carbohydrates: 11g

41. Tuna Salad

Preparation Time: 10 minutes
Cooking Time: none
Servings: 3
Ingredients :

- 1 can tuna (6 oz.)
- 1/3 cup fresh cucumber, chopped
- 1/3 cup fresh tomato, chopped
- 1/3 cup avocado, chopped

- 1/3 cup celery, chopped
- 2 garlic cloves, minced
- 4 tsp. olive oil
- 2 tbsp. lime juice
- Pinch of black pepper

Directions:
1. Prepare the dressing by combining olive oil, lime juice, minced garlic and black pepper.
2. Mix the salad **Ingredients** in a salad bowl and drizzle with the dressing.

Nutrition:

- Carbohydrates: 4.8 g
- Protein: 14.3 g
- Total sugars: 1.1 g
- Calories: 212 g

42. Roasted Portobello Salad

Preparation Time: 10 minutes
Cooking Time: none
Servings: 4
Ingredients :
- 11/2 lb. Portobello mushrooms, stems trimmed
- 3 heads Belgian endive, sliced
- 1 small red onion, sliced
- 4 oz. blue cheese
- 8 oz. mixed salad greens
- Dressing:
- 3 tbsp. red wine vinegar
- 1 tbsp. Dijon mustard
- 2/3 cup olive oil
- Salt and pepper to taste

Directions:

1. Preheat the oven to 450F.
2. Prepare the dressing by whisking together vinegar, mustard, salt and pepper. Slowly add olive oil while whisking.
3. Cut the mushrooms and arrange them on a baking sheet, stem-side up. Coat the mushrooms with some dressing and bake for 15 minutes.
4. In a salad bowl toss the salad greens with onion, endive and cheese. Sprinkle with the dressing.
5. Add mushrooms to the salad bowl.

Nutrition:

- Carbohydrates: 22.3 g
- Protein: 14.9 g
- Total sugars: 2.1 g, Calories: 501

43. Simple Deviled Eggs

Preparation Time: 5 minutes
Cooking Time: 8 minutes
Serving: 12
Ingredients :

- 6 large eggs
- 1/8 teaspoon mustard powder
- 2 tablespoons light mayonnaise

Direction:

1. Sit the eggs in a saucepan, then pour in enough water to cover the egg. Bring to a boil, then boil the eggs for another 8 minutes. Turn off the heat and cover, then let sit for 15 minutes.
2. Transfer the boiled eggs to a pot of cold water and peel under the water.
3. Transfer the eggs to a large plate, then cut in half. Remove the egg yolks and place them in a bowl, then mash with a fork.
4. Add the mustard powder, mayo, salt, and pepper to the bowl of yolks, then stir to mix well.
5. Spoon the yolk mixture in the egg white on the plate. Serve immediately.

Nutrition:

- 45 calories
- 1g carbohydrates
- 0.9g fiber

44. Sautéed Collard Greens and Cabbage

Preparation Time: 10 minutes
Cooking Time: 10 minutes
Serving: 8
Ingredients :

- 2 tablespoons extra-virgin olive oil
- 1 collard greens bunch
- ½ small green cabbage
- 6 garlic cloves
- 1 tablespoon low-sodium soy sauce

Direction:

1. Cook olive oil in a large skillet over medium-high heat.
2. Sauté the collard greens in the oil for about 2 minutes, or until the greens start to wilt.
3. Toss in the cabbage and mix well. Set to medium-low, cover, and cook for 5 to 7 minutes, stirring occasionally, or until the greens are softened.
4. Fold in the garlic and soy sauce and stir to combine. Cook for about 30 seconds more until fragrant.
5. Remove from the heat to a plate and serve.

Nutrition:

- 73 calories
- 5.9g carbohydrates
- 2.9g fiber

45. Roasted Delicata Squash with Thyme

Preparation Time: 10 minutes
Cooking Time: 20 minutes
Serving: 4
Ingredients :

- 1 (1½-pound) Delicata squash
- 1 tablespoon extra-virgin olive oil
- ½ teaspoon dried thyme
- ¼ teaspoon salt
- ¼ teaspoon freshly ground black pepper

Direction:

1. Prep the oven to 400°F (205°C). Ready baking sheet with parchment paper and set aside.
2. Add the squash strips, olive oil, thyme, salt, and pepper in a large bowl, and toss until the squash strips are fully coated.
3. Place the squash strips on the prepared baking sheet in a single layer. Roast for about 20 minutes, flipping the strips halfway through.
4. Remove from the oven and serve on plates.

Nutrition:

- 78 calories
- 11.8g carbohydrates
- 2.1g fiber

46. Roasted Asparagus and Red Peppers

Preparation Time: 5 minutes
Cooking Time: 15 minutes
Serving: 4
Ingredients :

- 1-pound (454 g) asparagus
- 2 red bell peppers, seeded
- 1 small onion
- 2 tablespoons Italian dressing

Direction:
1. Ready oven to (205°C). Wrap baking sheet with parchment paper and set aside.
2. Combine the asparagus with the peppers, onion, dressing in a large bowl, and toss well.
3. Arrange the vegetables on the baking sheet and roast for about 15 minutes. Flip the vegetables with a spatula once during cooking.
4. Transfer to a large platter and serve.

Nutrition:

- 92 calories
- 10.7g carbohydrates
- 4g fiber

47. Tarragon Spring Peas

Preparation Time: 10 minutes
Cooking Time: 12 minutes
Serving: 6
Ingredients :

- 1 tablespoon unsalted butter
- ½ Vidalia onion
- 1 cup low-sodium vegetable broth
- 3 cups fresh shelled peas
- 1 tablespoon minced fresh tarragon

Directions:
1. Cook butter in a pan at medium heat.
2. Sauté the onion in the melted butter for about 3 minutes, stirring occasionally.
3. Pour in the vegetable broth and whisk well. Add the peas and tarragon to the skillet and stir to combine.
4. Reduce the heat to low, cover, cook for about 8 minutes more, or until the peas are tender.
5. Let the peas cool for 5 minutes and serve warm.

- 82 calories
- 12g carbohydrates
- 3.8g fiber

48. Butter-Orange Yams

Preparation Time: 7 minutes
Cooking Time: 45 minutes
Serving: 8
Ingredients :

- 2 medium jewel yams
- 2 tablespoons unsalted butter
- Juice of 1 large orange
- 1½ teaspoons ground cinnamon
- ¼ teaspoon ground ginger
- ¾ teaspoon ground nutmeg
- 1/8 teaspoon ground cloves

Direction:

1. Set oven at 180°C.
2. Arrange the yam dices on a rimmed baking sheet in a single layer. Set aside.
3. Add the butter, orange juice, cinnamon, ginger, nutmeg, and garlic cloves to a medium saucepan over medium-low heat. Cook for 3 to 5 minutes, stirring continuously.
4. Spoon the sauce over the yams and toss to coat well.
5. Bake in the prepared oven for 40 minutes.
6. Let the yams cool for 8 minutes on the baking sheet before removing and serving.

Nutrition:

- 129 calories
- 24.7g carbohydrates
- 5g fiber

49. Roasted Tomato Brussels Sprouts

Preparation Time: 15 minutes
Cooking Time: 20 minutes
Serving: 4
Ingredients :

- 1-pound (454 g) Brussels sprouts
- 1 tablespoon extra-virgin olive oil
- ½ cup sun-dried tomatoes
- 2 tablespoons lemon juice
- 1 teaspoon lemon zest

Directions:

1. Set oven 205°C. Prep large baking sheet with aluminum foil.
2. Toss the Brussels sprouts in the olive oil in a large bowl until well coated. Sprinkle with salt and pepper.
3. Spread out the seasoned Brussels sprouts on the prepared baking sheet in a single layer.
4. Roast for 20 minutes, shake halfway through.
5. Remove from the oven then situate in a bowl. Whisk tomatoes, lemon juice, and lemon zest, to incorporate. Serve immediately.

Nutrition:

- 111 calories
- 13.7g carbohydrates
- 4.9g fiber

50. Lamb with Broccoli & Carrots

Preparation Time: 20 minutes
Cooking Time: 10 minutes
Servings: 4
Ingredients :

- 2 cloves garlic, minced
- 1 tablespoon fresh ginger, grated
- ¼ teaspoon red pepper, crushed
- 2 tablespoons low-sodium soy sauce

- 1 tablespoon white vinegar
- 1 tablespoon cornstarch
- 12 oz. lamb meat, trimmed and sliced
- 2 teaspoons cooking oil
- 1 lb. broccoli, sliced into florets
- 2 carrots, sliced into strips
- ¾ cup low-sodium beef broth
- 4 green onions, chopped
- 2 cups cooked spaghetti squash pasta

Directions:

1. Combine the garlic, ginger, red pepper, soy sauce, vinegar and cornstarch in a bowl.
2. Add lamb to the marinade.
3. Marinate for 10 minutes.
4. Discard marinade.
5. In a pan over medium heat, add the oil.
6. Add the lamb and cook for 3 minutes.
7. Transfer lamb to a plate.
8. Add the broccoli and carrots.
9. Cook for 1 minute.
10. Pour in the beef broth.
11. Cook for 5 minutes.
12. Put the meat back to the pan.
13. Sprinkle with green onion and serve on top of spaghetti squash.

Nutrition:

- Calories 205
- Total Fat 6 g
- Saturated Fat 1 g
- Cholesterol 40 mg
- Sodium 659 mg
- Total Carbohydrate 17 g

51. Rosemary Lamb

Preparation Time: 15 minutes
Cooking Time: 2 hours
Servings: 14
Ingredients :

- Salt and pepper to taste
- 2 teaspoons fresh rosemary, snipped
- 5 lb. whole leg of lamb, trimmed and cut with slits on all sides
- 3 cloves garlic, slivered
- 1 cup water

Directions:

1. Preheat your oven to 375 degrees F.
2. Mix salt, pepper and rosemary in a bowl.
3. Sprinkle mixture all over the lamb.
4. Insert slivers of garlic into the slits.
5. Put the lamb on a roasting pan.
6. Add water to the pan.
7. Roast for 2 hours.

Nutrition:

- Calories 136
- Total Fat 4 g
- Saturated Fat 1 g
- Cholesterol 71 mg
- Sodium 218 mg
- Protein 23 g
- Potassium 248 mg

Dinner

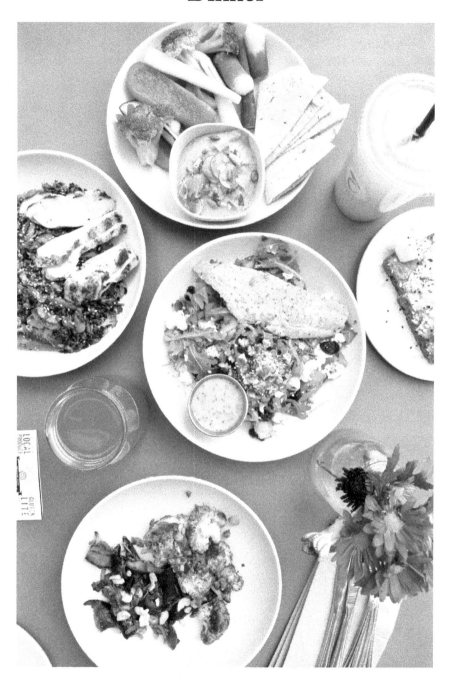

52. Tuna Sweet Corn Casserole

Preparation Time: 10 minutes
Cooking Time: 35 Minutes
Servings: 2
Ingredients :

- 3 small tins of tuna
- 0.5lb sweet corn kernels
- 1lb chopped vegetables
- 1 cup low sodium vegetable broth
- 2tbsp spicy seasoning

Directions:

1. Mix all the **Ingredients** in your Instant Pot.
2. Cook on Stew for 35 minutes.
3. Release the pressure naturally.

Nutrition:

- Calories: 300
- Carbs: 6
- Sugar: 1
- Fat: 9
- Protein:
- GL: 2

53. Lemon Pepper Salmon

Preparation Time: 10 minutes
Cooking Time: 10 Minutes
Servings: 4
Ingredients :

- 3 tbsps. ghee or avocado oil
- 1 lb. skin-on salmon filet
- 1 julienned red bell pepper
- 1 julienned green zucchini
- 1 julienned carrot
- ¾ cup water

- A few sprigs of parsley, tarragon, dill, basil or a combination
- 1/2 sliced lemon
- 1/2 tsp. black pepper
- ¼ tsp. sea salt

Directions:

1. Add the water and the herbs into the bottom of the Instant Pot and put in a wire steamer rack making sure the handles extend upwards.
2. Place the salmon filet onto the wire rack, with the skin side facing down.
3. Drizzle the salmon with ghee, season with black pepper and salt, and top with the lemon slices.
4. Close and seal the Instant Pot, making sure the vent is turned to "Sealing".
5. Select the "Steam" setting and cook for 3 minutes.
6. While the salmon cooks, julienne the vegetables, and set aside.
7. Once done, quick release the pressure, and then press the "Keep Warm/Cancel" button.
8. Uncover and wearing oven mitts, carefully remove the steamer rack with the salmon.
9. Remove the herbs and discard them.
10. Add the vegetables to the pot and put the lid back on.
11. Select the "Sauté" function and cook for 1-2 minutes.
12. Serve the vegetables with salmon and add the remaining fat to the pot.
13. Pour a little of the sauce over the fish and vegetables if desired.

Nutrition:

- Calories 296
- Carbs 8g
- Fat 15 g
- Protein 31 g
- Potassium (K) 1084 mg
- Sodium (Na) 284 mg

54. Chicken Zoodle Soup

Preparation Time: 15 minutes
Cooking Time: 35 minutes
Servings: 2
Ingredients :

- 1lb chopped cooked chicken
- 1lb spiralized zucchini
- 1 cup low sodium chicken soup
- 1 cup diced vegetables

Recipe:

1. Mix all the **Ingredients** except the zucchini in your Instant Pot.
2. Cook on Stew for 35 minutes.
3. Release the pressure naturally.
4. Stir in the zucchini and allow to heat thoroughly.

Nutrition:

- Calories: 250
- Carbs: 5
- Sugar: 0
- Fat: 10
- Protein: 40; GL: 1

55. Misto Quente

Preparation Time: 5 minutes
Cooking Time: 10 minutes
Servings: 4
Ingredients :

- 4 slices of bread without shell
- 4 slices of turkey breast
- 4 slices of cheese
- 2 tbsp. cream cheese
- 2 spoons of butter

Directions:
1. Preheat the air fryer. Set the timer of 5 minutes and the temperature to 200C.
2. Pass the butter on one side of the slice of bread, and on the other side of the slice, the cream cheese.
3. Mount the sandwiches placing two slices of turkey breast and two slices cheese between the breads, with the cream cheese inside and the side with butter.
4. Place the sandwiches in the basket of the air fryer. Set the timer of the air fryer for 5 minutes and press the power button.

Nutrition:

- Calories: 340
- Fat: 15g
- Carbohydrates: 32g
- Protein: 15g
- Sugar: 0g
- Cholesterol: 0mg

56. Garlic Bread

Preparation Time: 10 minutes
Cooking Time: 15 minutes
Servings: 4-5
Ingredients :
- 2 stale French rolls
- 4 tbsp. crushed or crumpled garlic
- 1 cup of mayonnaise
- Powdered grated Parmesan
- 1 tbsp. olive oil

Directions:
1. Preheat the air fryer. Set the time of 5 minutes and the temperature to 2000C.
2. Mix mayonnaise with garlic and set aside.
3. Cut the baguettes into slices, but without separating them completely.

4. Fill the cavities of equals. Brush with olive oil and sprinkle with grated cheese.
5. Place in the basket of the air fryer. Set the timer to 10 minutes, adjust the temperature to 1800C and press the power button.

Nutrition:

- Calories: 340
- Fat: 15g
- Carbohydrates: 32g
- Protein: 15g
- Sugar: 0g
- Cholesterol: 0mg

57. Bruschetta

Preparation Time: 5 minutes
Cooking Time: 10 minutes
Servings: 2
Ingredients :
- 4 slices of Italian bread
- 1 cup chopped tomato tea
- 1 cup grated mozzarella tea
- Olive oil
- Oregano, salt, and pepper
- 4 fresh basil leaves

Directions:
1. Preheat the air fryer. Set the timer of 5 minutes and the temperature to 2000C.
2. Sprinkle the slices of Italian bread with olive oil. Divide the chopped tomatoes and mozzarella between the slices. Season with salt, pepper, and oregano.
3. Put oil in the filling. Place a basil leaf on top of each slice.
4. Put the bruschetta in the basket of the air fryer being careful not to spill the filling. Set the timer of 5 minutes, set the temperature to 180C, and press the power button.
5. Transfer the bruschetta to a plate and serve.

Nutrition:

- Calories: 434
- Fat: 14g
- Carbohydrates: 63g
- Protein: 11g
- Sugar: 8g
- Cholesterol: 0mg

58. Cream Buns with Strawberries

Preparation Time: 10 minutes
Cooking Time: 12 minutes
Servings: 6
Ingredients :

- 240g all-purpose flour
- 50g granulated sugar
- 8g baking powder
- 1g of salt
- 85g chopped cold butter
- 84g chopped fresh strawberries
- 120 ml whipping cream
- 2 large eggs
- 10 ml vanilla extract
- 5 ml of water

Directions:

1. Sift flour, sugar, baking powder and salt in a large bowl. Put the butter with the flour with the use of a blender or your hands until the mixture resembles thick crumbs.
2. Mix the strawberries in the flour mixture. Set aside for the mixture to stand. Beat the whipping cream, 1 egg and the vanilla extract in a separate bowl.
3. Put the cream mixture in the flour mixture until they are homogeneous, and then spread the mixture to a thickness of 38 mm.
4. Use a round cookie cutter to cut the buns. Spread the buns with a combination of egg and water. Set aside

5. Preheat the air fryer, set it to 180C.
6. Place baking paper in the preheated inner basket.
7. Place the buns on top of the baking paper and cook for 12 minutes at 180C, until golden brown.

Nutrition:

- Calories: 150
- Fat: 14g
- Carbohydrates: 3g
- Protein: 11g
- Sugar: 8g
- Cholesterol: 0mg

59. Blueberry Buns

Preparation Time: 10 minutes
Cooking Time: 12 minutes
Servings: 6
Ingredients :

- 240g all-purpose flour
- 50g granulated sugar
- 8g baking powder
- 2g of salt
- 85g chopped cold butter
- 85g of fresh blueberries
- 3g grated fresh ginger
- 113 ml whipping cream
- 2 large eggs
- 4 ml vanilla extract
- 5 ml of water

Directions:

1. Put sugar, flour, baking powder and salt in a large bowl.
2. Put the butter with the flour using a blender or your hands until the mixture resembles thick crumbs.
3. Mix the blueberries and ginger in the flour mixture and set aside

4. Mix the whipping cream, 1 egg and the vanilla extract in a different container.
5. Put the cream mixture with the flour mixture until combined.
6. Shape the dough until it reaches a thickness of approximately 38 mm and cut it into eighths.
7. Spread the buns with a combination of egg and water. Set aside Preheat the air fryer set it to 180C.
8. Place baking paper in the preheated inner basket and place the buns on top of the paper. Cook for 12 minutes at 180C, until golden brown

Nutrition:

- Calories: 105
- Fat: 1.64g
- Carbohydrates: 20.09g
- Protein: 2.43g
- Sugar: 2.1g
- Cholesterol: 0mg

60. Cauliflower Potato Mash

Preparation Time: 30 minutes **Servings:** 4
Cooking Time: 5 minutes
Ingredients :
- 2 cups potatoes, peeled and cubed
- 2 tbsp. butter
- ¼ cup milk
- 10 oz. cauliflower florets
- ¾ tsp. salt

Directions:
1. Add water to the saucepan and bring to boil.
2. Reduce heat and simmer for 10 minutes.
3. Drain vegetables well. Transfer vegetables, butter, milk, and salt in a blender and blend until smooth.
4. Serve and enjoy.

Nutrition:

- Calories 128
- Fat 6.2 g
- Sugar 3.3 g
- Protein 3.2 g
- Cholesterol 17 mg

61. French toast in Sticks

Preparation Time: 5 minutes
Cooking Time: 10 minutes
Servings: 4
Ingredients :

- 4 slices of white bread, 38 mm thick, preferably hard
- 2 eggs
- 60 ml of milk
- 15 ml maple sauce
- 2 ml vanilla extract
- Nonstick Spray Oil
- 38g of sugar
- 3ground cinnamon
- Maple syrup, to serve
- Sugar to sprinkle

Directions:

1. Cut each slice of bread into thirds making 12 pieces. Place sideways
2. Beat the eggs, milk, maple syrup and vanilla.
3. Preheat the air fryer, set it to 175C.
4. Dip the sliced bread in the egg mixture and place it in the preheated air fryer. Sprinkle French toast generously with oil spray.
5. Cook French toast for 10 minutes at 175C. Turn the toast halfway through cooking.
6. Mix the sugar and cinnamon in a bowl.
7. Cover the French toast with the sugar and cinnamon mixture when you have finished cooking.
8. Serve with Maple syrup and sprinkle with powdered sugar

Nutrition:

- Calories 128
- Fat 6.2 g
- Carbohydrates 16.3 g
- Sugar 3.3 g
- Protein 3.2 g
- Cholesterol 17 mg

62. Muffins Sandwich

Preparation Time: 2 minutes
Cooking Time: 10 minutes
Servings: 1
Ingredients :

- Nonstick Spray Oil
- 1 slice of white cheddar cheese
- 1 slice of Canadian bacon
- 1 English muffin, divided
- 15 ml hot water
- 1 large egg
- Salt and pepper to taste

Directions:

1. Spray the inside of an 85g mold with oil spray and place it in the air fryer.
2. Preheat the air fryer, set it to 160C.
3. Add the Canadian cheese and bacon in the preheated air fryer.
4. Pour the hot water and the egg into the hot pan and season with salt and pepper.
5. Select Bread, set to 10 minutes.
6. Take out the English muffins after 7 minutes, leaving the egg for the full time.
7. Build your sandwich by placing the cooked egg on top of the English muffing and serve

Nutrition:

- Calories 400
- Fat 26g
- Carbohydrates 26g
- Sugar 15 g
- Protein 3 g
- Cholesterol 155 mg

63. Bacon BBQ

Preparation Time: 2 minutes
Cooking Time: 8 minutes
Servings: 2
Ingredients :

- 13g dark brown sugar
- 5g chili powder
- 1g ground cumin
- 1g cayenne pepper
- 4 slices of bacon, cut in half

Directions:

1. Mix seasonings until well combined.
2. Dip the bacon in the dressing until it is completely covered. Leave aside.
3. Preheat the air fryer, set it to 160C.
4. Place the bacon in the preheated air fryer
5. Select Bacon and press Start/Pause.

Nutrition:

- Calories: 1124
- Fat: 72g
- Carbohydrates: 59g
- Protein: 49g
- Sugar: 11g
- Cholesterol: 77mg

64. Stuffed French toast

Preparation Time: 4 minutes
Cooking Time: 10 minutes
Servings: 1
Ingredients :

- 1 slice of brioche bread,
- 64 mm thick, preferably rancid
- 113g cream cheese
- 2 eggs
- 15 ml of milk
- 30 ml whipping cream
- 38g of sugar
- 3g cinnamon
- 2 ml vanilla extract
- Nonstick Spray Oil
- Pistachios chopped to cover
- Maple syrup, to serve

Directions:

1. Preheat the air fryer, set it to 175C.
2. Cut a slit in the middle of the muffin.
3. Fill the inside of the slit with cream cheese. Leave aside.
4. Mix the eggs, milk, whipping cream, sugar, cinnamon, and vanilla extract.
5. Moisten the stuffed French toast in the egg mixture for 10 seconds on each side.
6. Sprinkle each side of French toast with oil spray.
7. Place the French toast in the preheated air fryer and cook for 10 minutes at 175C
8. Stir the French toast carefully with a spatula when you finish cooking.
9. Serve topped with chopped pistachios and acrid syrup.

Nutrition:

- Calories: 159
- Fat: 7.5g
- Carbohydrates: 25.2g
- Protein: 14g
- Sugar: 0g
- Cholesterol: 90mg

65. Scallion Sandwich

Preparation Time: 10 minutes
Cooking Time: 10 minutes
Servings: 1
Ingredients :

- 2 slices wheat bread
- 2 teaspoons butter, low fat
- 2 scallions, sliced thinly
- 1 tablespoon of parmesan cheese, grated
- 3/4 cup of cheddar cheese, reduced fat, grated

Directions:

1. Preheat the Air fryer to 356 degrees.
2. Spread butter on a slice of bread. Place inside the cooking basket with the butter side facing down.
3. Place cheese and scallions on top. Spread the rest of the butter on the other slice of bread Put it on top of the sandwich and sprinkle with parmesan cheese.
4. Cook for 10 minutes.

Nutrition:

- Calorie: 154
- Carbohydrate: 9g
- Fat: 2.5g
- Protein: 8.6g
- Fiber: 2.4g

66. Lean Lamb and Turkey Meatballs with Yogurt

Preparation Time: 10 minutes
Servings: 4
Cooking Time: 8 minutes
Ingredients :

- 1 egg white
- 4 ounces ground lean turkey
- 1 pound of ground lean lamb
- 1 teaspoon each of cayenne pepper, ground coriander, red chili pastes, salt, and ground cumin
- 2 garlic cloves, minced
- 1 1/2 tablespoons parsley, chopped
- 1 tablespoon mint, chopped
- 1/4 cup of olive oil

For the yogurt

- 2 tablespoons of buttermilk
- 1 garlic clove, minced
- 1/4 cup mint, chopped
- 1/2 cup of Greek yogurt, non-fat
- Salt to taste

Directions:

1. Set the Air Fryer to 390 degrees.
2. Mix all the **Ingredients** for the meatballs in a bowl. Roll and mold them into golf-size round pieces. Arrange in the cooking basket. Cook for 8 minutes.
3. While waiting, combine all the **Ingredients** for the mint yogurt in a bowl. Mix well.
4. Serve the meatballs with the mint yogurt. Top with olives and fresh mint.

Nutrition:

- Calorie: 154
- Carbohydrate: 9g
- Fat: 2.5g
- Protein: 8.6g
- Fiber: 2.4g

67. Air Fried Section and Tomato

Preparation Time: 10 minutes
Cooking Time: 5 minutes
Servings: 2
Ingredients :

- 1 aubergine, sliced thickly into 4 disks
- 1 tomato, sliced into 2 thick disks
- 2 tsp. feta cheese, reduced fat
- 2 fresh basil leaves, minced
- 2 balls, small buffalo mozzarella, reduced fat, roughly torn
- Pinch of salt
- Pinch of black pepper

Directions:

1. Preheat Air Fryer to 330 degrees F.
2. Spray small amount of oil into the Air fryer basket. Fry aubergine slices for 5 minutes or until golden brown on both sides. Transfer to a plate.
3. Fry tomato slices in batches for 5 minutes or until seared on both sides.
4. To serve, stack salad starting with an aborigine base, buffalo mozzarella, basil leaves, tomato slice, and 1/2-teaspoon feta cheese.
5. Top of with another slice of aborigine and 1/2 tsp. feta cheese. Serve.

Nutrition:

- Calorie: 140.3
- Carbohydrate: 26.6
- Fat: 3.4g
- Protein: 4.2g
- Fiber: 7.3g

68. Grain-Free Berry Cobbler

Preparation Time: 5 minutes
Cooking Time: 25 minutes
Servings: 10
Ingredients :

- 4 cups fresh mixed berries
- 1/2 cup ground flaxseed
- ¼ cup almond meal
- ¼ cup unsweetened shredded coconut
- 1/2 tablespoon baking powder
- 1 teaspoon ground cinnamon
- ¼ teaspoon salt
- Powdered stevia, to taste
- 6 tablespoons coconut oil

Directions:

1. Preheat the oven to 375F and lightly grease a 10-inch cast-iron skillet.
2. Spread the berries on the bottom of the skillet.
3. Whisk together the dry **Ingredients** in a mixing bowl.
4. Cut in the coconut oil using a fork to create a crumbled mixture.
5. Spread the crumble over the berries and bake for 25 minutes until hot and bubbling.
6. Cool the cobbler for 5 to 10 minutes before serving.

Nutrition:

- Calories 215
- Total Fat 16.8g
- Saturated Fat 10.4g
- Total Carbs 13.1
- Net Carbs 6.7g
- Protein 3.7g
- Sugar 5.3g
- Fiber 6.4g
- Sodium 61mg

69. Baked Salmon with Garlic Parmesan Topping

Preparation Time: 5 minutes,
Cooking Time: 20 minutes,
Servings: 4
Ingredients :

- 1 lb. wild caught salmon filets
- 2 tbsp. margarine
- What you'll need from store cupboard:
- ¼ cup reduced fat parmesan cheese, grated
- ¼ cup light mayonnaise
- 2-3 cloves garlic, diced
- 2 tbsp. parsley
- Salt and pepper

Directions:

1. Heat oven to 350 and line a baking pan with parchment paper.
2. Place salmon on pan and season with salt and pepper.
3. In a medium skillet, over medium heat, melt butter. Add garlic and cook, stirring 1 minute.
4. Reduce heat to low and add remaining **Ingredients** . Stir until everything is melted and combined.
5. Spread evenly over salmon and bake 15 minutes for thawed fish or 20 for frozen. Salmon is done when it flakes easily with a fork. Serve.

Nutrition:

- Calories 408
- Total Carbs 4g
- Protein 41g
- Fat 24g
- Sugar 1g
- Fiber 0g

70. Blackened Shrimp

Preparation Time: 5 minutes
Cooking Time: 5 minutes
Servings: 4
Ingredients :

- 1 1/2 lbs. shrimp, peel & devein
- 4 lime wedges
- 4 tbsp. cilantro, chopped
- What you'll need from store cupboard:
- 4 cloves garlic, diced
- 1 tbsp. chili powder
- 1 tbsp. paprika
- 1 tbsp. olive oil
- 2 tsp. Splenda brown sugar
- 1 tsp. cumin
- 1 tsp. oregano
- 1 tsp. garlic powder
- 1 tsp. salt
- 1/2 tsp. pepper

Directions:

1. In a small bowl combine seasonings and Splenda brown sugar.
2. Heat oil in a skillet over med-high heat. Add shrimp, in a single layer, and cook 1-2 minutes per side.
3. Add seasonings, and cook, stirring, 30 seconds. Serve garnished with cilantro and a lime wedge.

Nutrition:

- Calories 252
- Total Carbs 7g
- Net Carbs 6g
- Protein 39g
- Fat 7g
- Sugar 2g ; Fiber 1g

71. Cajun Catfish

Preparation Time: 5 minutes
Cooking Time: 15 minutes
Servings: 4
Ingredients :

- 4 (8 oz.) catfish fillets
- What you'll need from store cupboard:
- 2 tbsp. olive oil
- 2 tsp. garlic salt
- 2 tsp. thyme
- 2 tsp. paprika
- 1/2 tsp. cayenne pepper
- 1/2 tsp. red hot sauce
- ¼ tsp. black pepper
- Nonstick cooking spray

Directions:

1. Heat oven to 450 degrees. Spray a 9x13-inch baking dish with cooking spray.
2. In a small bowl whisk together everything but catfish. Brush both sides of fillets, using all the spice mix.
3. Bake 10-13 minutes or until fish flakes easily with a fork. Serve.

Nutrition:

- Calories 366
- Total Carbs 0g
- Protein 35g
- Fat 24g
- Sugar 0g
- Fiber 0g

72. Cajun Flounder & Tomatoes

Preparation Time: 10 minutes
Cooking Time: 15 minutes
Servings: 4
Ingredients :

- 4 flounder fillets
- 2 1/2 cups tomatoes, diced
- ¾ cup onion, diced
- ¾ cup green bell pepper, diced
- What you'll need from store cupboard:
- 2 cloves garlic, diced fine
- 1 tbsp. Cajun seasoning
- 1 tsp. olive oil

Directions:

1. Heat oil in a large skillet over med-high heat. Add onion and garlic and cook 2 minutes, or until soft. Add tomatoes, peppers and spices, and cook 2-3 minutes until tomatoes soften.
2. Lay fish over top. Cover, reduce heat to medium and cook, 5-8 minutes, or until fish flakes easily with a fork. Transfer fish to serving plates and top with sauce.

Nutrition:

- Calories 194
- Total Carbs 8g
- Net Carbs 6g
- Protein 32g
- Fat 3g
- Sugar 5g
- Fiber 2g

73. Cajun Shrimp & Roasted Vegetables

Preparation Time: 5 minutes
Cooking Time: 15 minutes
Servings: 4
Ingredients :

- 1 lb. large shrimp, peeled and deveined
- 2 zucchinis, sliced
- 2 yellow squash, sliced
- 1/2 bunch asparagus, cut into thirds
- 2 red bell pepper, cut into chunks
- What you'll need from store cupboard:
- 2 tbsp. olive oil
- 2 tbsp. Cajun Seasoning
- Salt & pepper, to taste

Directions:

1. Heat oven to 400 degrees.
2. Combine shrimp and vegetables in a large bowl. Add oil and seasoning and toss to coat.
3. Spread evenly in a large baking sheet and bake 15-20 minutes, or until vegetables are tender. Serve.

Nutrition:

- Calories 251
- Total Carbs 13g
- Net Carbs 9g
- Protein 30g
- Fat 9g
- Sugar 6g
- Fiber 4g

74. Cilantro Lime Grilled Shrimp

Preparation Time: 5 minutes,
Cooking Time: 5 minutes,
Servings: 6
Ingredients :

- 1 1/2 lbs. large shrimp raw, peeled, deveined with tails on
- Juice and zest of 1 lime
- 2 tbsp. fresh cilantro chopped
- What you'll need from store cupboard:
- ¼ cup olive oil
- 2 cloves garlic, diced fine
- 1 tsp. smoked paprika
- ¼ tsp. cumin
- 1/2 teaspoon salt
- ¼ tsp. cayenne pepper

Directions:

1. Place the shrimp in a large Ziploc bag.
2. Mix remaining **Ingredients** in a small bowl and pour over shrimp. Let marinate 20-30 minutes.
3. Heat up the grill. Skewer the shrimp and cook 2-3 minutes, per side, just until they turn pick. Be careful not to overcook them. Serve garnished with cilantro.

Nutrition:

- Calories 317 Total Carbs 4g Protein 39g Fat 15g Sugar 0g Fiber 0g

75. Crab Frittata

Preparation Time: 10 minutes
Cooking Time: 50 minutes
Servings: 4
Ingredients :

- 4 eggs
- 2 cups lump crabmeat
- 1 cup half-n-half
- 1 cup green onions, diced

- What you'll need from store cupboard:
- 1 cup reduced fat parmesan cheese, grated
- 1 tsp. salt
- 1 tsp. pepper
- 1 tsp. smoked paprika
- 1 tsp. Italian seasoning
- Nonstick cooking spray

Directions:
1. Heat oven to 350 degrees. Spray an 8-inch springform pan, or pie plate with cooking spray.
2. In a large bowl, whisk together the eggs and half-n-half. Add seasonings and parmesan cheese, stir to mix.
3. Stir in the onions and crab meat. Pour into prepared pan and bake 35-40 minutes, or eggs are set and top is lightly browned.
4. Let cool 10 minutes, then slice and serve warm or at room temperature.

Nutrition:

- Calories 276 Total
- Carbs 5g
- Net Carbs 4g
- Protein 25g
- Fat 17g
- Sugar 1g, Fiber 1g

76. Crunchy Lemon Shrimp

Preparation Time: 5 minutes
Cooking Time: 10 minutes,
Servings: 4
Ingredients :

- 1 lb. raw shrimp, peeled and deveined
- 2 tbsp. Italian parsley, roughly chopped
- 2 tbsp. lemon juice, divided
- What you'll need from store cupboard:
- 2/3 cup panko bread crumbs
- 2 1/2 tbsp. olive oil, divided
- Salt and pepper, to taste

Directions:
1. Heat oven to 400 degrees.
2. Place the shrimp evenly in a baking dish and sprinkle with salt and pepper. Drizzle on 1 tablespoon lemon juice and 1 tablespoon of olive oil. Set aside.
3. In a medium bowl, combine parsley, remaining lemon juice, bread crumbs, remaining olive oil, and ¼ tsp. each of salt and pepper. Layer the panko mixture evenly on top of the shrimp.
4. Bake 8-10 minutes or until shrimp are cooked through and the panko is golden brown.

Nutrition:

- Calories 283 Total Carbs 15g Net Carbs 14g Protein 28g Fat 12g Sugar 1g Fiber 1g

77. Grilled Tuna Steaks

Preparation Time: 5 minutes
Cooking Time: 10 minutes,
Servings: 6
Ingredients :

- 6 6 oz. tuna steaks
- 3 tbsp. fresh basil, diced
- What you'll need from store cupboard:
- 4 1/2 tsp. olive oil
- ¾ tsp. salt
- ¼ tsp. pepper
- Nonstick cooking spray

Directions:
1. Heat grill to medium heat. Spray rack with cooking spray.
2. Drizzle both sides of the tuna with oil. Sprinkle with basil, salt and pepper.
3. Place on grill and cook 5 minutes per side, tuna should be slightly pink in the center. Serve.

Nutrition:

- Calories 343 Total Carbs 0g Protein 51g Fat 14g Sugar 0g Fiber 0g

78. Red Clam Sauce & Pasta

Preparation Time: 10 minutes,
Cooking Time: 3 hours,
Servings: 4
Ingredients :

- 1 onion, diced
- ¼ cup fresh parsley, diced
- What you'll need from store cupboard:
- 2 6 1/2 oz. cans clams, chopped, undrained
- 14 1/2 oz. tomatoes, diced, undrained
- 6 oz. tomato paste
- 2 cloves garlic, diced
- 1 bay leaf
- 1 tbsp. sunflower oil
- 1 tsp. Splenda
- 1 tsp. basil
- 1/2 tsp. thyme
- 1/2 Homemade Pasta, cook & drain

Directions:

1. Heat oil in a small skillet over med-high heat. Add onion and cook until tender, add garlic and cook 1 minute more. Transfer to crock pot.
2. Add remaining **Ingredients** , except pasta, cover and cook on low 3-4 hours.
3. Discard bay leaf and serve over cooked pasta.

Nutrition:

- Calories 223
- Total Carbs 32g
- Net Carbs 27g
- Protein 12g
- Fat 6g
- Sugar 15g
- Fiber 5g

79. Salmon Milano

Preparation Time: 10 minutes,
Cooking Time: 20 minutes,
Servings: 6
Ingredients :

- 2 1/2 lb. salmon filet
- 2 tomatoes, sliced
- 1/2 cup margarine
- What you'll need from store cupboard:
- 1/2 cup basil pesto

Directions:

1. Heat the oven to 400 degrees. Line a 9x15-inch baking sheet with foil, making sure it covers the sides. Place another large piece of foil onto the baking sheet and place the salmon filet on top of it.
2. Place the pesto and margarine in blender or food processor and pulse until smooth. Spread evenly over salmon. Place tomato slices on top.
3. Wrap the foil around the salmon, tenting around the top to prevent foil from touching the salmon as much as possible. Bake 15-25 minutes, or salmon flakes easily with a fork. Serve.

Nutrition:

- Calories 444, Total Carbs 2g, Protein 55g, Fat 24g, Sugar 1g, Fiber 0g

80. Shrimp & Artichoke Skillet

Preparation Time: 5 minutes
Cooking Time: 10 minutes
Servings: 4
Ingredients :

- 1 1/2 cups shrimp, peel & devein
- 2 shallots, diced
- 1 tbsp. margarine
- What you'll need from store cupboard

- 2 12 oz. jars artichoke hearts, drain & rinse
- 2 cups white wine
- 2 cloves garlic, diced fine

Directions:
1. Melt margarine in a large skillet over med-high heat. Add shallot and garlic and cook until they start to brown, stirring frequently.
2. Add artichokes and cook 5 minutes. Reduce heat and add wine. Cook 3 minutes, stirring occasionally.
3. Add the shrimp and cook just until they turn pink. Serve.

Nutrition:

- Calories 487
- Total Carbs 26g
- Net Carbs 17g
- Protein 64g
- Fat 5g
- Sugar 3g
- Fiber 9g

81. Tuna Carbonara

Preparation Time: 5 minutes
Cooking Time: 25 minutes
Servings: 4
Ingredients :

- 1/2 lb. tuna fillet, cut in pieces
- 2 eggs
- 4 tbsp. fresh parsley, diced
- What you'll need from store cupboard:
- 1/2 Homemade Pasta, cook & drain,
- 1/2 cup reduced fat parmesan cheese
- 2 cloves garlic, peeled
- 2 tbsp. extra virgin olive oil
- Salt & pepper, to taste

Directions:
1. In a small bowl, beat the eggs, parmesan and a dash of pepper.
2. Heat the oil in a large skillet over med-high heat. Add garlic and cook until browned. Add the tuna and cook 2-3 minutes, or until tuna is almost cooked through. Discard the garlic.
3. Add the pasta and reduce heat. Stir in egg mixture and cook, stirring constantly, 2 minutes. If the sauce is too thick, thin with water, a little bit at a time, until it has a creamy texture.
4. Salt and pepper to taste and serve garnished with parsley.

Nutrition:

- Calories 409
- Total Carbs 7g
- Net Carbs 6g
- Protein 25g
- Fat 30g
- Sugar 3g
- Fiber 1g

82. Mediterranean Fish Fillets

Preparation Time: 10 minutes
Cooking Time: 3 minutes
Servings: 4
Ingredients :

- 4 cod fillets
- 1 lb. grape tomatoes, halved
- 1 cup olives, pitted and sliced
- 2 tbsp. capers
- 1 tsp. dried thyme
- 2 tbsp. olive oil
- 1 tsp. garlic, minced
- Pepper
- Salt

Directions:

1. Pour 1 cup water into the instant pot then place steamer rack in the pot.
2. Spray heat-safe baking dish with cooking spray.
3. Add half grape tomatoes into the dish and season with pepper and salt.
4. Arrange fish fillets on top of cherry tomatoes. Drizzle with oil and season with garlic, thyme, capers, pepper, and salt.
5. Spread olives and remaining grape tomatoes on top of fish fillets.
6. Place dish on top of steamer rack in the pot.
7. Seal pot with a lid and select manual and cook on high for 3 minutes.
8. Once done, release pressure using quick release. Remove lid.
9. Serve and enjoy.

Nutrition:

- Calories 212, Fat 11.9 g, Carbohydrates 7.1 g, Sugar 3 g, Protein 21.4 g, Cholesterol 55 mg

83. Garlic Sautéed Spinach

Preparation Time: 5 minutes
Cooking Time: 10 minutes
Servings: 4
Ingredients :

- 1 1/2 tablespoons olive oil
- 4 cloves minced garlic
- 6 cups fresh baby spinach
- Salt and pepper

Directions:

1. Heat the oil in a large skillet over medium-high heat.
2. Add the garlic and cook for 1 minute.
3. Stir in the spinach and season with salt and pepper.
4. Sauté for 1 to 2 minutes until just wilted. Serve hot.

Nutrition:

- Calories 60, Total Fat 5.5g
- Saturated Fat 0.8g, Total Carbs 2.6g
- Net Carbs 1.5g, Protein 1.5g
- Sugar 0.2g, Fiber 1.1g, Sodium 36mg

84. French Lentils

Preparation Time: 5 minutes
Cooking Time: 25 minutes
Servings: 10
Ingredients :
- 2 tablespoons olive oil
- 1 medium onion, diced
- 1 medium carrot, peeled and diced
- 2 cloves minced garlic
- 5 1/2 cups water
- 2 ¼ cups French lentils, rinsed and drained
- 1 teaspoon dried thyme
- 2 small bay leaves
- Salt and pepper

Directions:
1. Heat the oil in a large saucepan over medium heat.
2. Add the onions, carrot, and garlic and sauté for 3 minutes.
3. Stir in the water, lentils, thyme, and bay leaves – season with salt.
4. Bring to a boil then reduce to a simmer and cook until tender, about 20 minutes.
5. Drain any excess water and adjust seasoning to taste. Serve hot.

Nutrition:

- Calories 185, Total Fat 3.3g, Saturated Fat 0.5g
- Total Carbs 27.9g, Net Carbs 14.2g
- Protein 11.4g, Sugar 1.7g, Fiber 13.7g, Sodium 11mg

Dessert and Sweets

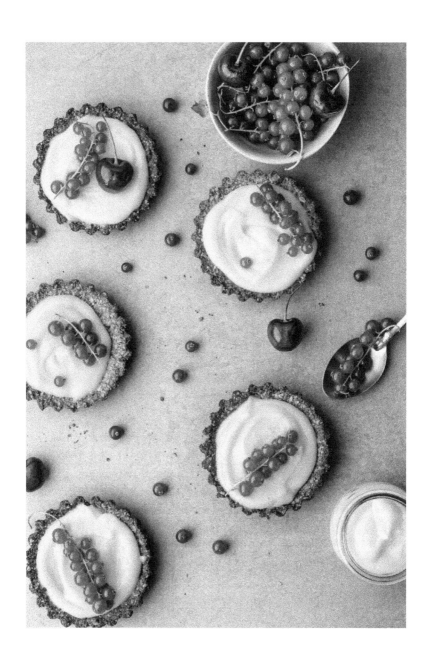

85. Frozen Lemon & Blueberry

Preparation Time: 5 minutes
Cooking Time: 10 minutes
Servings: 4
Ingredients :

- 6 cup fresh blueberries
- 8 sprigs fresh thyme
- ¾ cup light brown sugar
- 1 teaspoon lemon zest
- ¼ cup lemon juice
- 2 cups water

Directions:

1. Add blueberries, thyme and sugar in a pan over medium heat.
2. Cook for 6 to 8 minutes.
3. Transfer mixture to a blender.
4. Remove thyme sprigs.
5. Stir in the remaining **Ingredients** .
6. Pulse until smooth.
7. Strain mixture and freeze for 1 hour.

Nutrition:

- 78 Calories, 20g Carbohydrate, 3g Protein

86. Peanut Butter Choco Chip Cookies

Preparation Time: 5 minutes
Cooking Time: 10 minutes
Servings: 4
Ingredients :

- 1 egg
- ½ cup light brown sugar
- 1 cup natural unsweetened peanut butter
- Pinch salt
- ¼ cup dark chocolate chips

Directions:

1. Preheat your oven to 375 degrees F.
2. Mix egg, sugar, peanut butter, salt and chocolate chips in a bowl.
3. Form into cookies and place in a baking pan.
4. Bake the cookie for 10 minutes.
5. Let cool before serving.

Nutrition:

- 159 Calories
- 12g Carbohydrate
- 4.3g Protein

87. Watermelon Sherbet

Preparation Time: 5 minutes
Cooking Time: 3 minutes
Servings: 4
Ingredients :
- 6 cups watermelon, sliced into cubes
- 14 oz. almond milk
- 1 tablespoon honey
- ¼ cup lime juice
- Salt to taste

Directions:

1. Freeze watermelon for 4 hours.
2. Add frozen watermelon and other **Ingredients** in a blender.
3. Blend until smooth.
4. Transfer to a container with seal.
5. Seal and freeze for 4 hours.

Nutrition:

- 132 Calories
- 24.5g Carbohydrate
- 3.1g Protein

88. Strawberry & Mango Ice Cream

Preparation Time: 5 minutes
Cooking Time: 10 minutes
Servings: 4
Ingredients :

- 8 oz. strawberries, sliced
- 12 oz. mango, sliced into cubes
- 1 tablespoon lime juice

Directions:

1. Add all **Ingredients** in a food processor.
2. Pulse for 2 minutes.
3. Chill before serving.

Nutrition:

- 70 Calories
- 17.4g Carbohydrate
- 1.1g Protein

89. Sparkling Fruit Drink

Preparation Time: 5 minutes
Cooking Time: 10 minutes
Servings: 4
Ingredients :

- 8 oz. unsweetened grape juice
- 8 oz. unsweetened apple juice
- 8 oz. unsweetened orange juice
- 1 qt. homemade ginger ale
- Ice

Directions:

1. Makes 7 servings. Mix first 4 **Ingredients** together in a pitcher.
2. Stir in ice cubes and 9 ounces of the beverage to each glass.
3. Serve immediately.

Nutrition:

- 60 Calories
- 1.1g Protein

90. Tiramisu Shots
Preparation Time: 5 minutes
Cooking Time: 10 minutes
Servings: 4
Ingredients :

- 1 pack silken tofu
- 1 oz. dark chocolate, finely chopped
- ¼ cup sugar substitute
- 1 teaspoon lemon juice
- ¼ cup brewed espresso
- Pinch salt
- 24 slices angel food cake
- Cocoa powder (unsweetened)

Directions:

1. Add tofu, chocolate, sugar substitute, lemon juice, espresso and salt in a food processor.
2. Pulse until smooth.
3. Add angel food cake pieces into shot glasses.
4. Drizzle with the cocoa powder.
5. Pour the tofu mixture on top.
6. Top with the remaining angel food cake pieces.
7. Chill for 30 minutes and serve.

Nutrition:

- 75 Calories
- 12g Carbohydrate
- 2.9g Protein

91. Ice Cream Brownie Cake

Preparation Time: 5 minutes
Cooking Time: 10 minutes
Servings: 4
Ingredients :

- Cooking spray
- 12 oz. no-sugar brownie mix
- ¼ cup oil
- 2 egg whites
- 3 tablespoons water
- 2 cups sugar-free ice cream

Directions:

1. Preheat your oven to 325 degrees F.
2. Spray your baking pan with oil.
3. Mix brownie mix, oil, egg whites and water in a bowl.
4. Pour into the baking pan.
5. Bake for 25 minutes.
6. Let cool.
7. Freeze brownie for 2 hours.
8. Spread ice cream over the brownie.
9. Freeze for 8 hours.

Nutrition:
198 Calories
33g Carbohydrate
3g Protein

92. Peanut Butter Cups

Preparation Time: 5 minutes
Cooking Time: 10 minutes
Servings: 4
Ingredients :

- 1 packet plain gelatin
- ¼ cup sugar substitute
- 2 cups nonfat cream

- ½ teaspoon vanilla
- ¼ cup low-fat peanut butter
- 2 tablespoons unsalted peanuts, chopped

Directions:

1. Mix gelatin, sugar substitute and cream in a pan.
2. Let sit for 5 minutes.
3. Place over medium heat and cook until gelatin has been dissolved.
4. Stir in vanilla and peanut butter.
5. Pour into custard cups. Chill for 3 hours.
6. Top with the peanuts and serve.

Nutrition:
171 Calories
21g Carbohydrate; 6.8g Protein

93. Chocolate Avocado Mousse

Preparation Time: 10 minutes
Cooking Time: 5 minutes
Servings: 04
Ingredients :

- Coconut water, 2/3 cup
- Avocado, ½ hass
- Raw cacao, 2 teaspoons
- Vanilla, 1 teaspoon
- Dates, three (3)
- Sea salt, One (1) teaspoon
- Dark chocolate shavings

Directions:

1. Blend all **Ingredients** .
2. Blast until it becomes thick and smooth, as you wish.
3. Put in a fridge and allow it to get firm.

Nutrition:

- Calories: 181.8; Fat: 151. g; Protein: 12 g

94. Chia Vanilla Coconut Pudding

Preparation Time: 5 minutes
Cooking Time: 5 minutes
Servings: 2
Ingredients :

- Coconut oil, 2 tablespoons
- Raw cashew, ½ cup
- Coconut water, ½ cup
- Cinnamon, 1 teaspoon
- Dates (pitted), 3
- Vanilla, 2 teaspoons
- Coconut flakes (unsweetened), 1 teaspoon
- Salt (Himalayan or Celtic Grey)
- Chia seeds, 6 tablespoons
- Cinnamon or pomegranate seeds for garnish (optional)

Directions:

1. Get a blender, add all the **Ingredients** (minus the pomegranate and chia seeds), and blend for about forty to sixty seconds.
2. Reduce the blender speed to the lowest and add the chia seeds.
3. Pour the content into an airtight container and put in a refrigerator for five to six hours.
4. To serve, you can garnish with the cinnamon powder of pomegranate seeds.

Nutrition:

- Calories: 201
- Fat: 10 g
- Sodium: 32.8 mg

95. Sweet Tahini Dip with Ginger Cinnamon Fruit

Preparation Time: 10 minutes
Cooking Time: 5 minutes
Servings: 2
Ingredients :

- Cinnamon, one (1) teaspoon
- Green apple, one (1)
- Pear, one (1)
- Fresh ginger, two (2) – three (3)
- Celtic sea salt, one (1) teaspoon
- Ingredient for sweet Tahini
- Almond butter (raw), three (3) teaspoons
- Tahini (one big scoop), three (3) teaspoons
- Coconut oil, two (2) teaspoons
- Cayenne (optional), ¼ teaspoons
- Wheat-free tamari, two (2) teaspoons
- Liquid coconut nectar, one (1) teaspoon

Directions:
1. Get a clean mixing bowl.
2. Grate the ginger, add cinnamon, sea salt and mix together in the bowl.
3. Dice apple and pear into little cubes, turn into the bowl and mix.
4. Get a mixing bowl and mix all the **Ingredients** .
5. Then add the Sprinkle the Sweet Tahini Dip all over the Ginger Cinnamon Fruit.
6. Serve.

Nutrition:

- Calories: 109
- Fat: 10.8 g
- Sodium: 258 mg

96. Coconut Butter and Chopped Berries with Mint

Preparation Time: 5 minutes
Cooking Time: 5 minutes
Servings: 04
Ingredients :
- Chopped mint, one (1) tablespoon
- Coconut butter (melted), two (2) tablespoons
- Mixed berries (strawberries, blueberries, and raspberries)

Directions:
1. Get a small bowl and add the berries.
2. Drizzle the melted coconut butter and sprinkle the mint.
3. Serve.

Nutrition:

- Calories: 159, Fat: 12 g, Carbohydrates: 18 g

97. Alkaline Raw Pumpkin Pie

Preparation Time: 5 minutes
Cooking Time: 5 minutes
Servings: 04
Ingredients :
Ingredients for Pie Crust
- Cinnamon, one (1) teaspoon
- Dates/Turkish apricots, one (1) cup
- Raw almonds, one (1) cup
- Coconut flakes (unsweetened), one (1) cup

Ingredients for Pie Filling
- Dates, six (6)
- Cinnamon, ½ teaspoon
- Nutmeg, ½ teaspoon
- Pecans (soaked overnight), one (1) cup
- Organic pumpkin Blends (12 oz.), 1 ¼ cup
- Nutmeg, ½ teaspoon
- Sea salt (Himalayan or Celtic Sea Salt), ¼ teaspoon
- Vanilla, 1 teaspoon
- Gluten-free tamari

Directions:

Directions for pie crust
1. Get a food processor and blend all the pie crust **Ingredients** at the same time.
2. Make sure the mixture turns oily and sticky before you stop mixing.
3. Put the mixture in a pie pan and mold against the sides and floor, to make it stick properly.

Directions for the pie filling
1. Mix **Ingredients** together in a blender.
2. Add the mixture to fill in the pie crust.
3. Pour some cinnamon on top.
4. Then refrigerate till it's cold.
5. Then mold.

Nutrition:

- Calories 135, Calories from Fat 41.4.
- Total Fat 4.6 g, Cholesterol 11.3 mg

98. Strawberry Sorbet

Preparation Time: 5 minutes
Cooking Time: 4 Hours
Servings: 4
Ingredients :

- 2 cups of Strawberries*
- 1 1/2 teaspoons of Spelt Flour
- 1/2 cup of Date Sugar
- 2 cups of Spring Water

Directions:

1. Add Date Sugar, Spring Water, and Spelt Flour to a medium pot and boil on low heat for about ten minutes. Mixture should thicken, like syrup.
2. Remove the pot from the heat and allow it to cool.
3. After cooling, add Blend Strawberry and mix gently.
4. Put mixture in a container and freeze.

5. Cut it into pieces, put the sorbet into a processor and blend until smooth.
6. Put everything back in the container and leave in the refrigerator for at least four hours.
7. Serve and enjoy your Strawberry Sorbet!

Nutrition:

- Calories: 198, Carbohydrates: 28 g

99. Blueberry Muffins

Preparation Time: 5 minutes
Cooking Time: 1 Hour
Servings: 3
Ingredients :
- 1/2 cup of Blueberries
- 3/4 cup of Teff Flour
- 3/4 cup of Spelt Flour
- 1/3 cup of Agave Syrup
- 1/2 teaspoon of Pure Sea Salt
- 1 cup of Coconut Milk
- 1/4 cup of Sea Moss Gel (optional, check information)
- Grape Seed Oil

Directions:
1. Preheat your oven to 365 degrees Fahrenheit.
2. Grease or line 6 standard muffin cups.
3. Add Teff, Spelt flour, Pure Sea Salt, Coconut Milk, Sea Moss Gel, and Agave Syrup to a large bowl. Mix them together.
4. Add Blueberries to the mixture and mix well.
5. Divide muffin batter among the 6 muffin cups.
6. Bake for 30 minutes until golden brown.
7. Serve and enjoy your Blueberry Muffins!

Nutrition:

- Calories: 65, Fat: 0.7 g
- Carbohydrates: 12 g, Protein: 1.4 g, Fiber: 5 g

100.   Banana Strawberry Ice Cream

Preparation Time: 5 minutes
Cooking Time: 4 Hours
Servings: 5
Ingredients :

- 1 cup of Strawberry*
- 5 quartered Baby Bananas*
- 1/2 Avocado, chopped
- 1 tablespoon of Agave Syrup
- 1/4 cup of Homemade Walnut Milk

Directions:
1. Mix **Ingredients** into the blender and blend them well.
2. Taste. If it is too thick, add extra Milk or Agave Syrup if you want it sweeter.
3. Put in a container with a lid and allow to freeze for at least 5 to 6 hours.
4. Serve it and enjoy your Banana Strawberry Ice Cream!

Nutrition:

- Calories: 200, Fat: 0.5 g, Carbohydrates: 44 g

101.   Homemade Whipped Cream

Preparation Time: 5 minutes
Cooking Time: 10 Minutes
Servings: 1 Cup
Ingredients :

- 1 cup of Aquafaba
- 1/4 cup of Agave Syrup

Directions:
1. Add Agave Syrup and Aquafaba into a bowl.
2. Mix at high speed around 5 minutes with a stand mixer or 10 to 15 minutes with a hand mixer.
3. Serve and enjoy your Homemade Whipped Cream!

Nutrition:

- Calories: 21, Fat: 0g, Sodium: 0.3g
- Carbohydrates: 5.3g, Fiber: 0g, Sugars: 4.7g, Protein: 0g

Conclusion

Type 1 diabetes is all about being proactive, and being able to recognize when your blood sugars are getting too high and when they're too low. There are a lot of people with type 1 diabetes who don't know when their blood sugars are too high or too low or in what range they should be. Type II diabetes is the more common form of diabetes. It accounts for about 90 percent of diabetes cases. Type II diabetes usually occur because a person's body has lost the ability to produce insulin.

Type 1 diabetes occurs because the immune system destroys the insulin-producing cells of the pancreas. In the early stages of the disease, you may experience episodes of low blood sugar, called hypoglycemia, that can be dangerous if they occur frequently.

Having Type 1 diabetes will teach you a load of tough lessons. Only about ¼ of diabetics are Type 1. But I'm here to tell you, even though Type 1 is the most common type of diabetes, Type 2 diabetes can be almost as bad.

Being diagnosed with the disease will bring some major changes in your lifestyle. From the time you are diagnosed with it, it would always be a constant battle with food. You need to become a lot more careful with your food choices and the quantity that you ate. Every meal will feel like a major effort. You will be planning every day for the whole week, well in advance. Depending upon the type of food you ate, you have to keep checking your blood sugar levels. You may get used to taking long breaks between meals and staying away from snacks between dinner and breakfast.

Food would be treated as a bomb like it can go off at any time. According to an old saying, "When the body gets too hot, then your body heads straight to the kitchen."

Managing diabetes can be a very, very stressful ordeal. There will be many times that you will mark your glucose levels down on a piece of paper like you are plotting graph lines or something. You will mix your insulin shots up and then stress about whether or not you are giving yourself the right dosage. You will always be over-cautious because it involves a LOT of math and a really fine margin of error. But now, those days are gone!

With the help of technology and books, you can stock your kitchen with the right foods, like meal plans, diabetic friendly dishes, etc. You can get an app that will even do the work for you. You can also people-watch on the internet and find the know-how to cook and eat right; you will always be a few meals away from certain disasters, like a plummeting blood sugar level. Always carry some sugar in your pocket. You won't have to experience the pangs of hunger but if you are unlucky, you will have to ration your food and bring along some simple low-calorie snacks with you.

As you've reached the end of this book, you have gained complete control of your diabetes and this is just the beginning of your journey towards a better, healthier life.

Regardless of the length or seriousness of your diabetes, it can be managed! Take the information presented here and start with it!

Lightning Source UK Ltd.
Milton Keynes UK
UKHW021845100621
385314UK00002B/306